PON

Also by the American Cancer Society
Colorectal Cancer
Prostate Cancer

American Cancer Society
WOMEN AND CANCER

American Cancer Society

WOMEN AND CANCER

A Thorough and Compassionate Resource for Patients and Their Families

Carolyn D. Runowicz, M.D.,
Jeanne A. Petrek, M.D.,
and
Ted S. Gansler, M.D.

Editorial Project Director
Dianne Partie Lange

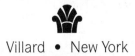

Villard • New York

ISBN 0-679-77814-4

Random House website address: www.atrandom.com

Printed in the United States of America on acid-free paper

98765432

First Edition

Contents

1. Cancer in Women   3

Part I   The Breast

2. The Healthy Breast   19
3. What Is Breast Cancer?   36
4. Risk Factors   41
5. Diagnosis   52
6. If the Diagnosis Is Cancer   66
7. Surgery   86
8. Radiation Therapy   119
9. Chemotherapy   126

Part II   The Cervix

10. The Healthy Cervix   147
11. Who Is at Risk?   158
12. Precancerous Conditions   162
13. When the Diagnosis Is Cancer   167
14. Treatment   171

Part III   The Uterus

15. The Healthy Uterus   *183*
16. Diagnosis and Staging   *190*
17. Treatment of Endometrial Cancer   *197*

Part IV   The Ovaries

18. The Healthy Ovary   *205*
19. Is It Ovarian Cancer?   *215*
20. Treatment of Ovarian Cancer   *223*
21. Life after Cancer   *232*
    Appendix   *243*
    Resources   *245*
    Index   *265*

American Cancer Society
WOMEN AND CANCER

Chapter 1

Cancer in Women

If you have recently been told that you have cancer, or if someone close to you has just heard the news, you are being challenged emotionally as well as physically. You need answers to many questions, ranging from the most basic and general—"What is cancer?"—to the more specific and uniquely personal—"What is the best treatment for *me?*" Doctors who specialize in treating women who have cancer agree that learning about the disease is an important first step toward wellness and healing. When some of the mystery of the disease can be eliminated, the stress you feel can be alleviated and you can learn what you need to know to make smart choices about your treatment.

Each section of *Women and Cancer* is devoted to one of the four female organs in which cancer most often develops: the breast, the cervix, the uterus, and the ovaries. The initial chapter in each section describes the organ's structure (anatomy) and how it functions (physiology). Learning how your body works when it is healthy will help you understand the impact of cancer and the effects that various treatments will have, particularly if surgery is required. There are many myths and misunderstandings about the effects of surgery on a woman's sexual and reproductive organs. It's important that you know the facts.

Following each section's brief and basic lesson in anatomy and physiology are: a description of the diagnostic tests you may be given, and a discussion of how your physician can determine exactly what type of cancer you have. This information will prepare you for the sometimes tedious diagnostic process and will help you to understand why your doctors recommend certain tests instead of others, and why some testing may be repeated. You will learn what tests are available. You can then pursue alternatives that may not be initially offered in conjunction with your diagnosis. Throughout the book, you will be reminded that not all cancers are alike, even when they are found in a particular organ. The type of breast cancer a relative or friend had may be very different—in its growth rate or extent of spread for instance—than the tumor just diagnosed in your breast.

Each section concludes with a discussion of the treatments that are usually recommended: surgery, radiation, chemotherapy, and, in some cases, hormone therapy. How these treatments and their possible side effects—short-term and long-term, transient and permanent—will affect your life is described realistically.

In Section I, breast cancer, the most common cancer of female organs, is discussed in great detail. Read this section, regardless of the type of cancer you are dealing with. It contains important information about how malignancy develops in any part of the body, the various means designed to obliterate a malignancy. The information in the breast cancer section is cross-referenced, rather than duplicated, in the other sections of the book. For instance, the side effects of chemotherapy are similar, whether a woman is receiving the anticancer drugs for ovarian cancer or breast cancer. If your primary concern is ovarian cancer, refer to the breast cancer section to learn how to cope with the side effects of chemotherapy.

Cancers of the cervix, uterus, and ovaries are the most common cancers of the female reproductive system. More unusual

There is so much pressure to feel positive. You feel it from your family, your friends, the outside world. It's great that lots of women are surviving and living longer, but there is this quality that you can't have a negative thought . . . that negative thoughts are bad for you. There is the suggestion that negative thoughts are how you got the disease in the first place. I'm not sure that people really believe that, but there is the suggestion of it. It's hard to keep pushing that suggestion away. You tell yourself, "No, it's not true. I didn't bring this upon myself."

—J.C.

cancers, and cancers that have spread to the reproductive system from other organs, are not discussed in this book. Nevertheless, because the treatments for these cancers are very similar, the information given here may prove helpful. For more specific information, contact the American Cancer Society at 800-ACS-2345 or check its Web site at www.cancer.org.

This book is meant to guide you through the cancer treatment process and to help you ask the right questions when you are discussing your personal issues with your doctor. The information is organized to fill in the gaps of your understanding of cancer, but keep in mind that this is a general overview of several cancers that are unique to women and that the condition, its treatment, and response for yourself, or someone you care for, are unique.

THE TRUTH IS IN THE NUMBERS

Sometimes it seems as though there's a cancer epidemic. Everyone you talk to knows someone—and often is very close to someone—who has recently been diagnosed with the disease. Heart

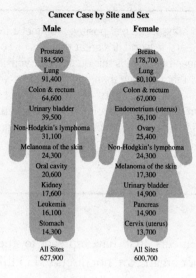

Cancer Case by Site and Sex

Male	Female
Prostate 184,500	Breast 178,700
Lung 91,400	Lung 80,100
Colon & rectum 64,600	Colon & rectum 67,000
Urinary bladder 39,500	Endometrium (uterus) 36,100
Non-Hodgkin's lymphoma 31,100	Ovary 25,400
Melanoma of the skin 24,300	Non-Hodgkin's lymphoma 24,300
Oral cavity 20,600	Melanoma of the skin 17,300
Kidney 17,600	Urinary bladder 14,900
Leukemia 16,100	Pancreas 14,900
Stomach 14,300	Cervix (uterus) 13,700
All Sites 627,900	All Sites 600,700

Cancer Deaths by Site and Sex

Male	Female
Lung 93,100	Lung 67,000
Prostate 39,200	Breast 43,500
Colon & rectum 27,900	Colon & rectum 28,600
Pancreas 14,000	Pancreas 14,900
Non-Hodgkin's lymphoma 13,000	Ovary 14,500
Leukemia 12,000	Non-Hodgkin's lymphoma 11,900
Esophagus 9,100	Leukemia 9,600
Urinary bladder 8,400	Endometrium (uterus) 6,300
Stomach 8,100	Brain 6,000
Liver 7,900	Stomach 5,000
All Sites 294,200	All Sites 270,600

*Excluding basal and squamous cell skin cancer and in situ carcinomas except urinary bladder.
American Cancer Society, Surveillance Research, 1998.
© 1998, American Cancer Society, Inc.

Figure 1.1: Leading sites of new cancer cases and deaths—1998 estimates. *

disease is the number-one killer of American women, but cancer seems to be their greatest fear.

Annually, about 1,228,600 people are diagnosed as having a malignancy. This figure does not include noninvasive cancer, known as carcinoma in situ, and it omits basal and squamous cell skin cancers, of which over one million cases are diagnosed each year.

In 1992, the incidence rate of cancer in the United States began to decline after decades of escalation. The death rate from cancer is also declining: between 1991 and 1995, the national cancer death rate fell 2.6 percent. This is probably because of fewer deaths from malignancies that begin in the lung, colon–rectum, and prostate in men; and in the breast, colon-rectum, and gynecologic sites in women. Cancer is responsible for one of every four deaths in the United States, but it's important to keep in mind that more Americans than ever are cancer survivors. About eight million living Americans now have a history of cancer.

Lung, colorectal, breast, and prostate cancers are the leading causes of deaths from cancer in the United States. In 1987, lung cancer became the number-one killer of both men and women, and it remains in that lead position in 1998. In women, deaths from lung cancer are followed by those from breast cancer, cancer of the colon and rectum, and pancreatic cancer. (In Europe, breast cancer death rates remain higher than deaths from lung cancer.)

BREAST CANCER

Breast cancer accounts for about one of every three cancer diagnoses among women. Excluding cancer of the skin, breast cancer is the most common cancer in the United States. For four decades, the incidence of breast cancer had been rising; in the 1990s, it appears to be stabilizing. It is now estimated that one in every eight women in the developed world will get breast cancer in her lifetime. (Breast cancer in men is rare; in 1998, about 1,600 new cases were diagnosed in American men.)

Experts link the increased number of breast cancer cases diagnosed during the late 1980s to more widespread use of mammography, a screening test that allows cancer to be discovered even before a tumor can be felt. After any screening test becomes common practice, the incidence of cases rises for several years, because more cancers are being detected. Eventually, the annual statistics on new cases stabilize. Before widespread screening with mammography, breast cancers were discovered only after they had grown large enough to cause signs or symptoms, such as a lump that could be felt. With mammography, cancers that are too small to be felt can be found, along with symptomatic cancers. Were it not for screening, those small cancers may not have been found until they were considerably enlarged, several years later.

Other sources continue to contribute to the general rise in incidence of breast cancer. Some scientists suspect that our increasingly polluted environment—and particularly our exposure to pesticides—is partly at fault, but, thus far, scientific studies have not confirmed this concern. In fact, in 1997, a study on a possible link between environmental contaminants and breast cancer risk suggested that exposure to organochlorines in pesticides and industrial chemicals (DDT and PCBs,* for example) does not increase breast cancer risk. Other scientists believe that the trend toward delaying pregnancy is partially responsible for

* DDT = dichlor-diphenyl-trichloride; PCBs = polychlorinated biphenyls.

the increase, and some blame changes in women's nutritional habits and lack of physical activity.

There is a decline in mortality from breast cancer, particularly among White and African American women under age fifty. This trend may be due to improvements in breast cancer treatment— that is, the increased use of chemotherapy—and to mammography screening, which allows breast cancers to be diagnosed at an earlier stage.

Interpreting Risk

If the statistics on breast cancer are startling, it may be helpful to put them in perspective. Consider this: less than 4 percent of American women will die of breast cancer while about 30 percent will die from heart disease. This statistical comparison has been used to counsel women on the benefits of estrogen replacement therapy, which is helpful in preventing heart disease but may increase the risk of breast cancer.

The numbers cited in statistical statements can be confusing. For example, in 1993, when women learned that their lifetime risk of developing breast cancer had increased from one in nine to one in eight (12.5%), many were understandably concerned about the new, very grim statistic. The numbers are correct, but it's important to know that "lifetime" risk describes the risk that a *girl just born* will develop breast cancer during the course of *her* lifetime. For a woman in her forties, fifties, or sixties, the risk of developing breast cancer in the next ten years is defined by a quite different set of numbers (see Table 1.1).

The odds of developing breast cancer are increased if a woman's mother or sister has been diagnosed with breast cancer. If her first-degree relative was under age fifty at the time of diagnosis, the woman's risk is 13 to 21 percent. If the relative was over

TABLE 1.1: WOMEN'S AGE AND THE PROBABILITY OF DEVELOPING BREAST CANCER		
Current Age (Years)	Probability of Developing Breast Cancer in the Next Ten Years	or 1 in
20	0.04%	2,500
30	0.40	250
40	1.49	67
50	2.54	39
60	3.43	29

fifty, the risk is 9 to 11 percent. If a woman's mother *and* sister were diagnosed with breast cancer when they were under age fifty, the risk to the woman is 35 to 48 percent. If both first-degree relatives were over fifty, the risk is 11 to 24 percent.

CANCERS OF THE REPRODUCTIVE ORGANS

The female reproductive system includes the cervix, endometrium (the lining of the upper part of the uterus), and ovaries. When cancer in any of these organs is detected early, the possibility of cure is good. For each type of cancer, the five-year relative survival rate is better than 90 percent when the disease is detected early. Cancer of the cervix can be detected early by means of a Pap test (see Chapter 11). Unfortunately, there are no screening tests that indicate an early cancer is present in the ovaries or in the endometrium, so detection may not occur until the disease creates noticeable symptoms. Therefore, it's extremely important for women to be alert to any signs or symptoms of abnormal function—unusual bleeding, pelvic or abdominal tenderness or pain, or bloating—and to see a gynecologist annually for a pelvic exam.

Cancer of the Endometrium

The incidence rate of cancer of the endometrium has been relative constant since the late 1980s, when an estimated 21 cases per 100,000 women were diagnosed each year. About 36,100 cases of cancer of the uterus were diagnosed in 1998, and most of those originated in the endometrium, the most common site of gynecologic cancer.

Mortality rates of endometrial cancer have also been relatively constant at about 3 per 100,000 per year. About 6,300 women died of this cancer during 1998. Like cancer of the ovary, the only routine screening test for endometrial cancer is a pelvic examination in which the physician palpates the uterus. Rarely is this type of malignancy detected at an early stage by a Pap test. However, because symptoms such as vaginal bleeding after menopause or irregular periods typically prompt a woman to see a doctor, endometrial cancer can usually be detected at an early stage.

Cancer of the Ovary

Cancer of one of the two ovaries, the egg- and hormone-producing organs of the female reproductive system, ranks second among gynecologic cancers. In 1998, about 25,400 new cases of ovarian cancer were diagnosed. About one in fifty-five or about 2 percent of American women will develop ovarian cancer during her lifetime. If a woman's mother or sister has ovarian cancer, her risk is 5 percent; if two first-degree relatives have ovarian cancer, the woman's risk is 7 percent.

In 1998, about 14,500 American women died of ovarian cancer. This malignancy causes more deaths than any other cancer of the reproductive system, and it is the fifth leading cause of all cancer deaths in women. Ovarian cancer is so lethal because it tends to be already advanced when it is diagnosed. The signs and symptoms of ovarian cancer are often subtle. And, many of these symptoms, such as nausea, bloating and constipation are often attributed to benign digestive system problems.

The only routine screening test is a pelvic examination in which the doctor palpates the ovaries, which may not change detectably until the cancer is advanced. Another factor is that many women do not have routine exams.

If diagnosed and treated early, the survival rate is 92 percent. However, only about one in four ovarian cancers is diagnosed at this early stage.

Cancer of the Cervix

Cancer of the cervix, the narrow neck of the uterus that projects into the upper third of the vagina, is the third most common female reproductive system cancer and the second most common cause of death from gynecologic malignancy. An estimated 13,700 cases of invasive cancer were diagnosed in 1998. Carcinoma in situ is diagnosed much more frequently, particularly in women under fifty. (Remember that carcinoma in situ is noninvasive and is quite responsive to treatment. Women with this stage of the disease are not included in the above estimate.)

There is evidence that preinvasive cervical cancer can progress to invasive cancer, but early preinvasive lesions may also do the opposite and spontaneously regress. Fortunately, the incidence of invasive cervical cancer has been decreasing steadily, as has the death rate from the disease. Since the introduction of screening with the Pap test (see Chapter 10), the mortality rate from cervical cancer is estimated to have declined about 70 percent. In fact, because cervical cancer can remain preinvasive for a long time—during which it can be effectively treated—it is considered by many experts to be a preventable cancer. Still, there is much room for improvement. In 1998, about 4,900 women died of invasive cervical cancer.

THE CHALLENGE OF CANCER

Cancer is a group of many diseases, all caused by the abnormal growth of cells. This overproduction of cells is the result of a change in genetic information. You may have been born with a particular genetic alteration or, more likely, you may have developed it during your life.

Normal cells reproduce themselves in a process called cell division, and at some genetically predetermined point, they die. When certain changes in the cell's genetic material cause it to become malignant, the offspring of that cell not only fail to die on schedule, but they also often replicate themselves more than is normal. The result is an accumulation of abnormal cells. This overgrowth of cells forms a tumor, and some of the cells may invade normal tissues, often interfering with the functioning ability of the organ they have invaded. Malignant cells also may enter the bloodstream and lymphatic vessels and travel (metastasize) to distant sites, where the cells continue to proliferate.

In each of the sections that follow, you will learn how cancer affects the female organ in which a tumor forms, and what steps can be taken to get rid of the tumor and any wayward cancer cells. You will also learn that cancer cells vary enormously in their aggressiveness (how quickly the cells grow and how likely they are to spread).

Whether the organ involved is the breast, an ovary, the cervix, or the endometrium, cancer treatment almost always begins with surgery, unless the cancer is far advanced and/or a woman is in

SCREENING TESTS

A screening test is a test or examination given at specific intervals to people who have no symptoms of cancer, in an effort to detect the disease at an early stage. The American Cancer Society recommends the following procedures for women:

Site	*Recommendation*
General cancer-related checkup	Every three years for women ages twenty to forty, and every year for those forty and older. The checkup should include health counseling and, depending on a woman's age, might include examination for cancer of the thyroid, skin, oral cavity, lymph nodes, and ovaries.
Breast	For women age forty and older: Annually, a mammogram and a clinical breast exam, performed by a health care professional, close to the scheduled mammogram; monthly, a breast self-examination. For women ages twenty to thirty-nine: a clinical breast exam every three years and a monthly self-examination.
Colon and rectum	Women age fifty and older should follow one of these examination schedules:

- A fecal occult blood test every year and a flexible sigmoidoscopy every five years.

- A colonoscopy every ten years.

- A double-contrast barium enema every five to ten years.

- A digital rectal exam, done at the same time as the sigmoidoscopy, colonoscopy, or double-contrast barium enema.

Women who are at moderate or high risk for colorectal cancer should talk with a doctor about a different testing schedule.

Uterus

Cervix: All women who are or have been sexually active or who are age eighteen and older should have an annual Pap test and pelvic examination. After three or more consecutive satisfactory examinations with normal findings, the Pap test may be performed less frequently. Discuss with your physician the schedule that is best for you.

such poor health that she is not a good surgical candidate. Chemotherapy or radiation therapy may then be offered prior to surgery or in place of it.

In the past, surgeons treating breast cancer thought it was necessary to remove the entire breast and perhaps some surrounding tissues in order to successfully treat the disease. Now, many studies have shown that removing the lump with a margin of normal breast tissue may be the only surgical treatment necessary. This operation is called a lumpectomy.

New methods of treating abnormal cells on the cervix are helping many women avoid removal of the uterus (hysterectomy), thus preserving their ability to have children. A hysterectomy is not always needed to treat ovarian cancer in young women.

Other aspects of treatment—*radiation*, which destroys cancer cells in the targeted area, and *chemotherapy*, which affects rapidly dividing cancer cells throughout the body—continue to be the mainstay of therapy when malignancy has spread beyond the original or *primary* tumor. New drugs and new combinations of standard drugs are constantly being evaluated. Today, some drugs—such as tamoxifen (Nolvadex)—are prescribed as preventives against cancer recurrence. Studies have indicated that tamoxifen can reduce the recurrence of breast cancer by as much as 45 percent.

As you read about the types of reproductive cancers and their treatments, you may be surprised to learn that there is an enormously varied menu of possibilities and options. Your physician will offer the therapy plan believed to be most effective in treating your particular type and stage of cancer. There may be options within the plan, based on your general health, your age, and your life situation. Some choices are clear; other decisions are more complex. If you seek a second opinion, another doctor may suggest other possible options. This book will give you a foundation for understanding what you need to know about cancer and will help you to ask the right questions, enabling you to participate actively in your own care.

Part I
The Breast

Chapter 2

The Healthy Breast

Unlike any other organ of a woman's body, the breasts are both a visible symbol of femininity and a functioning glandular system. Breast size is partially an inherited trait, but whether they are large or small, pendulous or firm, a woman's breasts affect her self-image. They are a barometer of hormonal and weight changes, and they respond visibly to sexual stimulation. Breasts are not critical to life but, throughout a woman's life, they herald certain changes in her physiology.

Considering the attention breast cancer has received in recent years, even women who have never been particularly conscious of changes in their breasts can't escape being aware that they are also a common site for a life-threatening malignancy. Understanding how your breasts function, how they feel, and how they respond to your hormonal ebbs and flows, may help you to detect signs of potential problems. Should any abnormal condition develop, whether benign or malignant, knowing the basics of your own anatomy can help you make wise decisions about what to do.

BREASTS AND HORMONES

In girls, breast tissue is present from birth, but the breasts begin changing noticeably in puberty. The increased production of female hormones prompts a cascade of physical changes that herald the transition from child to woman. There's an increase in fatty breast tissue, which determines the size and shape of the breasts; the nipples, and the areolas that surround them, enlarge. The breasts are typically symmetrical, but it is not unusual for the left breast to be slightly larger than the right.

Breasts are milk-producing and milk-secreting glands. During puberty, estrogen and other hormones stimulate the growth of

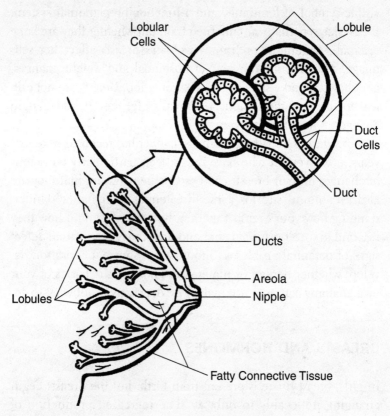

Figure 2.1: Breast structure.

epithelial cells. As a young girl matures, these cells develop to form a network of lobules. The whole process takes several years and, at times, the breasts may be quite tender. Figure 2.1 shows the breast structure.

Each *mammary gland* is a collection of fifteen to twenty lobes. Each lobe is made up of twenty to forty even smaller lobules. Small saclike units, not unlike a cluster of grapes, form each *lobule*. The lobules open into small *ducts* or tubes that join progressively larger ducts. Underneath the areola in each breast, the ducts meet in reservoirs called *milk sinuses*. From there, canals extend through each nipple and open onto its surface.

Mammary ligaments, also called *Cooper's ligaments*, extend from the bottommost layer of skin covering each breast to the pectoralis muscle of the chest wall beneath it. These ligaments hold the breasts in place on top of the chest, aligned over the third to the sixth (or seventh) rib. Some breast tissue extends from the top of the breasts outward toward the underarm areas. Over time, the ligaments supporting the breasts may stretch, depending on the weight of the tissue they contain and the number of times a woman is pregnant. Blood vessels weave throughout this network of fat, glands, muscles, and ligaments. Arteries supply the breast tissue with fresh, oxygen-laden blood, and veins carry the oxygen-depleted blood and waste products away. Each breast is also supplied with nerve fibers, which extend from branches of major nerves in the chest (see Figure 2.2). *Lymphatic vessels* carry tissue fluid called *lymph* to *lymph nodes* where the fluid is filtered. The lymph nodes contain immune system cells that will recognize any germs in the lymph, and help fight the infection. Small lymphatic vessels within the breast tissue join together into larger vessels. Most of these vessels lead to lymph nodes under the arms (*axillary nodes*), but some lead to lymph nodes beneath the breastbone (*sternum*). Breast cancer cells sometimes enter the lymphatic vessels and may spread to these lymph nodes.

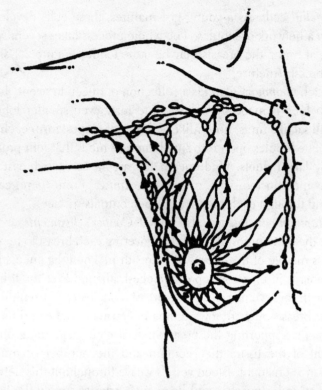

Figure 2.2: Lymphatic vessels of the breast and underarm area.

HOW BREASTS CHANGE THROUGHOUT A WOMAN'S LIFE

When you began to menstruate regularly, your breasts underwent fairly predictable cycles. Before ovulation, when an ovary is being stimulated to produce an egg by follicle-stimulating hormone (FSH), estrogen is released and circulates to all the tissues of your body, including those in the breast, where the hormone stimulates cell growth. In the middle of the cycle, luteinizing hormone (LH) causes the ovary to release an egg from a follicle. The follicle then begins producing progesterone, which increases blood flow to the breast, causing its veins to fill with more blood than usual. During this premenstrual time, the amount of tissue fluid within the breast increases, and some women complain that their breasts feel swollen and are especially tender or sensitive.

If pregnancy doesn't occur, the newly formed breast cells die and are absorbed by the body. But if the egg is fertilized, the lobules of the breast continue to develop. The epithelial cells grown and mature, or *differentiate*, as the glandular system of the breast prepares to perform its biological function—to make milk. Within about two months, the areola and nipple of each breast will darken—another characteristic early sign of pregnancy.

Immediately before the birth of a child, lactation or milk production begins. As milk is secreted by the glands, the breasts enlarge, stretching the tissue covering them and the ligaments that support them. Tiny bumps on each areola, which are a kind of oil gland, secrete a natural lubricant to keep the nipples supple during breast feeding. When the mother stops nursing the infant, the glands within the breast return to nearly the size they were before pregnancy, and the excess breast cells die and are absorbed by the body. However, there is always some permanent change in the breasts. Most often, the breasts will soften and droop a bit as a result of the stretching. The nipple and areola usually lighten again but do not return to their previous color.

After menopause, when the hormonal stimulation becomes erratic and finally ceases, the breasts develop an even smoother, softer quality. The milk-producing apparatus is no longer active, so the glands shrink. Dense breast tissue is gradually replaced by fat, and the breasts tend to droop even more. Hormone replacement may arrest or slow this process, and exercise that develops the chest muscles beneath the breasts may make them appear more prominent, but some degree of sagging is inevitable as a woman ages.

Throughout the course of your life—particularly if you practice monthly self-examination—you will become familiar with all the cyclic changes in your breasts and the "feel" of your unique combination of glandular and fatty tissue. You will know whether a certain amount of lumpiness in your breasts is normal for you, and you will become familiar enough with this texture to detect an unusual change that needs to be checked by your doctor.

Women have three basic exams available to *screen* or detect abnormalities that may indicate cancer: (1) mammography, an X-ray of the breast; (2) clinical breast examination (CBE) by a physician or a nurse; and (3) breast self-examination (BSE).

MAMMOGRAPHY

A mammogram is a low-dose breast X-ray. It serves as a screening test for women who have no symptoms of breast cancer and as a strategic test for women who have discovered an abnormal lump (see Chapter 6).

The American Cancer Society recommends that women have a yearly mammogram beginning at age forty. A mammogram is advised in addition to BSE and CBE because it is capable of detecting lumps that are too small to feel. In 76 to 94 percent of women who have a malignancy, mammography will reveal the cancer. That is not to say a mammogram is foolproof. If a distinct, solid lump is felt and a mammogram is negative, a biopsy is still necessary for an accurate diagnosis (see Chapter 6). On average, mammography has about a 15 percent failure rate—that is, it fails to diagnose a cancer that is present. Because the breasts of

> The thought had crossed my mind that I might have breast cancer,
> but then I thought, "No, it's not going to be. I'm going to be OK."
> Since I had had eight operations for bone infection and two artificial
> knees, I thought, "I've had my share." But the Lord had a different out-
> look on things. I do have faith. I believe in prayer, and I think that is a
> big help. When I found it was cancer, I just said, "You gave it to me,
> Lord, you get me through it." I have a very optimistic outlook on
> things, so that's the way I went into it. I can beat this thing.
>
> —J. S.

young women are dense and can be difficult to visualize on an
X-ray, the failure rate of mammography is higher in young
women and lower in older ones.

The Controversy over Recommendations

It has long been known that women age fifty and over benefit
from annual mammography, but there is much debate regarding whether the breast X-ray is effective enough in women
under fifty to warrant its widespread use as a screening test. The
American Medical Association, the American College of Obstetrics and Gynecology, the American Women's Medical Association, the National Medical Association, and the American
Society of Radiology agree with the American Cancer Society's
recommendation for women in their forties. Organizations
that advise mammography only for women fifty and over include the American Academy of Family Practice, the American
College of Physicians, and the United States Preventive Services Task Force.

Recently, several conferences of health care professionals and related organizations have yielded differing guidelines on mammography for women in their forties. In an effort to resolve the controversy, eight randomized, controlled trials are being conducted in different countries to determine whether screening mammography is effective in women under age fifty. These studies began between 1963 and 1982 and require a long follow-up period to evaluate whether fewer deaths occur from breast cancer in the screened versus the nonscreened group. The results at ten to twelve years indicated a 16 percent decrease in mortality in the screened group. The actual benefit to women in 1998 is expected to be higher.

Although they are significant, these ongoing studies may be underestimating the benefit of early mammography, for four reasons.

1. They may not have included enough women in their forties.
2. Some women assigned to the mammography screening group did not receive the test, and some assigned to the control group received mammograms outside the study.
3. Some participants are being screened every two years, which spaces the tests too far apart for detecting fast-growing cancers.
4. The technology for doing breast X-rays has improved in the past fifteen years.

Today, mammography is able to detect cancers that are smaller and at earlier stages than those that could be detected on an X-ray in the past. Remember that the earlier cancer is detected, the greater is the likelihood that the woman will survive at least five to ten years.

Mammography's assistance in detecting cancer in women over fifty has never been questioned. According to the National

Cancer Institute/American Cancer Society Breast Cancer Detection Demonstration Project, a 30 percent reduction in breast cancer deaths was realized in women over fifty who had both a CBE and a mammogram every year.

Having a Mammogram

A mammography machine is an X-ray machine with a device that compresses the breast between two square plastic plates (Figure 2.3). The image that results is two-dimensional. Two X-rays are taken of each breast: one from above and another from the side.

The flatter the breast, the more accurate the image, and the machine's pressure on the breast can be uncomfortable. But the X-ray takes only a few minutes, and most women are able to tolerate the discomfort. If possible, schedule a mammogram when your breasts are least sensitive — usually, a week after the start of your menstrual period. Some women have extremely sensitive breasts, and researchers have found that by allowing these women to control the pressure of the plates themselves, a good mammogram can be accomplished. To keep your chest still, you will be asked to hold your breath for the few seconds during which the X-ray is actually taken.

PREPARING FOR YOUR MAMMOGRAM

The night or morning before your mammogram appointment, shower or bathe to remove any trace of powder, deodorant, or anything else that might show up on the X-ray. If past mammograms have been painful for you, try avoiding caffeine during the week before the test. You will be asked to remove any jewelry from your neck, so you might as well leave any chains or necklaces at home.

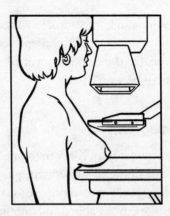

Figure 2.3: The X-ray machine for mammography.

After the X-ray is completed, the film must be reviewed, to be sure the image is not blurred. If it's not clear, or if a radiologist is present and notices anything that arouses immediate concern, more X-rays may be taken. You may be called back in a few days, if the films have been examined and more views are needed for diagnostic reasons.

Some women are concerned about the radiation exposure associated with any X-ray. Advances in mammography have made the radiation exposure minimal.

The radiologist may tell you the result based on a quick look at your X-ray before you leave the facility, but a more careful reading will be done later and the results will be sent to your physician in a written report. You can ask to have a copy sent to you as well.

Keeping a Record

When a mammogram shows something abnormal, your doctor may want to compare it to a prior mammogram, so it's important to keep track of when and where your earlier breast X-rays were done. Alternatively, you can keep the actual X-ray films yourself. The most important thing is to have the test regularly. For older women, one way to remember an annual mammogram is to make the appointment on your birthday—a date you aren't likely to forget.

CLINICAL BREAST EXAMINATION

A clinical breast examination (CBE) is done by a health professional—a doctor, nurse practitioner, or nurse. The American Cancer Society recommends that every woman between the ages of twenty and thirty-nine should have a CBE at least every three years. Starting at age forty, a woman should have a CBE annually even when she has an annual mammogram, so that the information from the two tests can be integrated. Sometimes, a palpable breast lump (a lump that can be felt) may not appear on a mammogram but a doctor or nurse may discover it when doing a CBE.

The examiner will first look at your breasts, to note any changes in their shape or size, or any signs of nipple inversion or

---

AMERICAN CANCER SOCIETY GUIDELINES FOR BREAST CANCER DETECTION

Breast Self-Examination (BSE):
Age twenty or over—every month.

Clinical Breast Examination (CBE):
Age twenty to forty—every three years.
Age forty or over—every year.

Mammography:
Age forty or over—every year.

skin dimpling. Then he or she will palpate your breasts and feel your chest area and armpits, searching for lumps. The doctor or nurse is trained to notice any abnormalities in breast texture. If a lump is found, he or she will note its size, precisely where it's located, how hard it feels, and whether it's attached to the skin or to deeper tissues.

A CBE is done both while you are lying flat and when you are in an upright position. You may also be asked to sit and bend forward while the appearance of your breasts is checked. The examiner may occasionally also tug or squeeze your nipples to see if fluid is expressed.

BREAST SELF-EXAMINATION

The American Cancer Society recommends that women age twenty and older practice monthly breast self-examination (BSE). By examining your own breasts at regular intervals, you are more likely to find changes that occur between the times when you have CBEs or mammograms. Women who do regular BSE are more likely to notice changes early rather than to discover problems by chance.

In recent years, questions have been raised about the value of BSE for extending life if a change turns out to be breast cancer. A few studies have concluded that BSE does not improve survival time but many researchers feel that flaws in the way the studies were designed or carried out make these conclusions unreliable. To date, no studies proving routine BSE does improve the chances of surviving breast cancer have been done. Nevertheless, the American Cancer Society considers routine, monthly BSE to be an opportunity to discover breast cancer early, when it is most likely to be responsive to treatment.

Most women find the BSE procedure more comfortable, and their breasts less bumpy, in the week following the start of their menstrual period. At this time, breasts are softer, and any change in their texture is easier to notice. Other women—especially those who do not have regular periods, or are pregnant, or no longer menstruate—find it's easiest to remember to do BSE on a fixed schedule: the first of the month, or perhaps the first Saturday of each month. If you are nursing, do your BSE when you are finished with a feeding.

The procedure is simple. (Step-by-step instructions are given in the box on pages 32–35.) If you are unsure about how to feel or *palpate* your breasts, ask your doctor or a nurse to teach you the technique. Gynecologists and women's health centers often have videotapes that show how to examine the breasts with the flat part of the fingertips, and some doctors even have models— complete with abnormal lumps—on which you can practice.

If you have never done BSE, it may take several months for you to learn what is normal for you. One way to know whether something is normal is to check if you feel something similar on the opposite breast. If you are doing BSE for the first time, ask your doctor or nurse to show you have and then repeat exactly what he or she has just done. This is a good time to ask whether what you're feeling is normal.

Another way to "memorize" the normal texture of your own breasts is to practice examining yourself every day for ten days following a CBE by a health care professional. After you are familiar with how your healthy breast feels, you are more likely to detect subtle changes. You may even be able to note changes that your doctor—who examines your breast once a year—doesn't feel.

Finding a lump, feeling unusual tenderness or pain, or noticing redness or secretion from a nipple may be a sign that something unusual is happening in your breast, but these symptoms do not always indicate a malignancy. Many other conditions can cause a change in breast texture. For example, a new or unusual mass may be a *cyst*—a harmless, fluid-filled sac. Lobules sometimes form benign solid lumps known as *fibroadenomas*. Some women's breasts tend to be more lumpy, or *fibrocystic*, and this

---

HOW TO DO BREAST SELF-EXAMINATION

As you feel each breast, notice whether there are any changes in the usual texture of your breast tissue. Are there any lumps or tender areas? As you look at your breasts, are there any signs of irritation (redness), puckering of the skin, or unusual asymmetry? Do you notice any secretions from the nipple?

1. Lie down, and place a pillow under your right shoulder, to help flatten your right breast. Place your right arm behind your head. (If your breasts are large, you may want to use your right hand to hold your breast while you examine it with your left hand.)

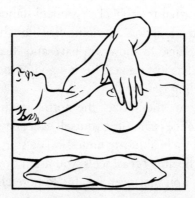

2. Use the finger pads of the three middle fingers on your left hand to feel for lumps in the right breast. (A finger pad is the top third of each finger.)

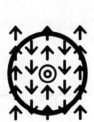
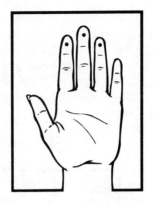

3. Press firmly enough to know how your breast feels. It's helpful to vary the pressure, from light to deep, with each palpation. A firm ridge in the lower curve of the bottom of each breast is normal.

4. Move your finger pads around the breast in a set way. You can choose to move your finger pads up and down in vertical strips, around in a circle, or from the outside toward the center in a wedge pattern, but be sure to do it the same way every time.

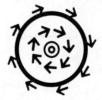

   Go over the entire breast and chest area. The chest area extends from the middle of the armpit to just beneath the breast, across the underside of the breast to the middle of the breastbone, up along the breastbone to the collarbone, and back to the middle of the armpit.

5. With your arm relaxed at your side, examine the breast tissue that extends into your armpit.

6. Repeat the exam on your left breast, using the finger pads of your right hand.
7. Repeat the exam standing up. With your left arm raised and your left hand behind your head, examine your left breast with your right hand by repeating steps 2 through 5.
8. During a shower or bath, you might want to repeat the BSE. Your soapy hands gliding over the wet skin will make it easy to check the breasts' texture.

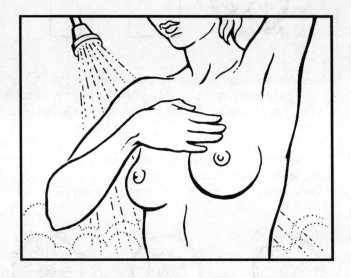

9. If you find any changes, call and tell your doctor what you have noticed, and ask for an appointment.
10. For added safety, you may want to check your breasts as you stand in front of a mirror. Stand with your arms relaxed at your sides. Look for any changes in the breasts' (and the nipples') appearance, including dimpling of the skin, redness, or swelling. Continue standing and repeat the visual examination with your hands on your hips, and then with your arms raised above your head while you lean forward.

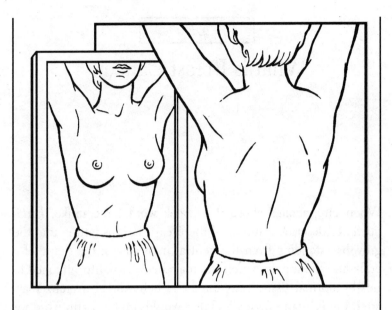

11. Although some nipple discharge occurs normally in premenopausal women, report any secretions to your doctor, regardless
of your age.

condition may be painful. Infections can occur in the breasts,
causing tenderness and inflammation. This is particularly common in nursing women. The skin over the breasts can become irritated and dry. Sometimes, the breasts may actually secrete fluid.
All of these conditions are considered benign and may or may not
require treatment or further testing (see Chapter 5).

Chapter 3

What Is Breast Cancer?

When Hippocrates chose the Greek word for crablike, *karki-noma*, to describe a tumor of the breast, he was noting that the growths extending from the central mass gave it the shape of a crab, and the way in which the mass became tightly attached to nearby normal tissue resembled the behavior of a crab. Years later, the Roman physician Galen would use the Latin word for crab, *cancer*, to describe such masses. Both physicians were well aware of the life-threatening nature of the disease. In those ancient times, primitive attempts were made to remove malignant breast tumors without benefit of anesthesia. Occasionally, the treatment worked, provided the woman survived the operation, but more often than not, the cancer returned. Many more centuries passed before scientists would begin to understand that cancer is a disease of altered cells and molecules, and before doctors could effectively treat this disease.

Cancer is really a group of many related diseases rather than one single disease. These diseases share many features, but also have important differences, because they develop in different organs and from different types of cells. Most cancers in humans begin in the *epithelial cells*, the cells that line the body's internal surfaces, including the glands. A cancer that originates in the epithelial cells is called a *carcinoma*. When cancer affects the epithelial cells of a gland—as happens in breast, stomach, and intestinal cancers, among others—it is called an *adenocarcinoma*.

CELL REPLICATION

If you could peer into a cell through a microscope so powerful that it allowed you to see the individual chemical molecules in the cellular "soup," you would see that the basis of life is unique combinations of four *nucleotides*: adenine, thymine, cytosine, and guanine. Certain sequences of these chemicals—called genes—are linked end-to-end in each of two strands that form the double helix of deoxyribonucleic acid, better known as DNA. Long, tightly coiled strands of DNA make a chromosome, and each cell has forty-six of them.

Every time a cell divides, the threads of DNA inside each chromosome separate into two strands, and an identical copy of each strand is made within the cell. Each of the two new daughter cells will have an identical set of matching chromosomes, including the DNA they contain, provided there have been no mistakes in the copying process—no accidents, no injuries, and no mutations in the genes. Normally, cell replication is regulated to match the number of cells that wear out and die. Sometimes, this well-orchestrated turnover cycle goes awry. Too many cells form, because their growth is too rapid and not properly controlled.

In any tissue of the body, this overproduction of cells is called hyperplasia. When it occurs in the breast ducts, it is called *ductal hyperplasia*; if it occurs in the lobules, it's *lobular hyperplasia*. If these excess cells have an abnormal appearance, the condition is further described as *atypical hyperplasia*. If the cells are not atypical, the diagnosis is *usual hyperplasia*. It's important to understand that none of these conditions is cancer. In fact, ductal or lobular hyperplasia may exist for years and never cause any problems. Furthermore, atypical cells may revert to normal. If growth of the atypical cells becomes quite extensive, the condition is referred to as *ductal carcinoma in situ*, or *lobular carcinoma in situ*, depending on whether the cells are developing within the ducts or the lobules.

INVASIVE CANCER

What happens next—if the situation progresses at all—is that the malformed cells of *carcinoma in situ* do not stay within a duct or lobule, but continue to multiply and eventually break through the wall of the duct or lobe and invade surrounding tissue. This condition is called *invasive* or *infiltrating breast cancer*.

Although cancer cells may take years to form a detectable tumor, a mass will eventually form. The cancer will also stimulate the growth of nearby blood vessels in a process known as *angiogenesis*. The blood vessels help the cancer continue to grow by providing it with additional oxygen and nutrients.

Often, the larger the cancer becomes, the more likely it will invade healthy surrounding tissues, including the walls of blood and lymphatic vessels. A *benign* tumor, in contrast, does not invade into neighboring tissues or *metastasize* (spread to other organs). Benign tumors in some organs can grow large enough to put pressure on nearby tissue and organs.

When cancer cells extend beyond the primary site and invade the muscle beneath the breast, *local spread* has occurred. When cancer cells enter the lymphatic vessels and spread to the axillary lymph nodes, it is referred to as *regional spread* or *lymph node metastasis*.

Once cancer cells have access to the bloodstream or the lymphatic system, they can travel to distant parts of the body. If they are not destroyed by the person's immune system, they begin forming additional tumors in other organs. At this point, the situation is described as *distant spread* or *distant metastasis*. If it involves a vital organ like the lungs or the brain and is not treated, or fails to respond to treatment, it may eventually prevent that organ from performing life-supporting functions. When people die of breast cancer, it is because of metastases to vital organs.

Generally, the larger a cancer is, the more likely it has spread to other organs, which is why so much emphasis is on detecting cancer early, when the tumor is still small and more likely to be curable. However, there are exceptions to this generalization. For example, some small tumors can be *aggressive*: they are likely to spread to the regional lymph nodes and metastasize throughout the body. This is why, when breast cancer of any size is diagnosed, the surgeon usually examines some of the lymph nodes under the arm to check for signs of invasion. Aggressive breast cancer is more common in younger women. Breast tumors may also be slow-growing. Some can remain localized within a breast for many years.

When a breast lump is removed, a pathologist examines it under a microscope, looking for any traits that may indicate that it is aggressive. These *prognostic factors* are discussed in Chapter 5.

> I have a very optimistic outlook on things, so that's the way I went into it. I can beat this thing. There is life after breast cancer, I'm sure . . . . I don't want to dwell on the negative aspects of it. It happened; I had no control over it happening, but I do have control over what happens after it.
>
> —J.S.

THE BODY FIGHTS BACK

If you're a healthy person with an active immune system, your body doesn't allow these wayward cells to grow out of control without notice. The immune system goes on alert when it detects any invaders, including the body's own abnormal cells. Disease-fighting cells of the immune system circulate in the bloodstream and continually attempt to ferret out and destroy cancer cells. In fact, some experts believe that cells capable of becoming invasive cancer are always present, but the body's immune system is able to destroy them. Whether cancer gains a foothold in the body because it overwhelms the normal disease-fighting mechanisms or whether the immune system is inhibited by unknown forces has not been determined. Scientists do know that poor nutrition, inactivity, poor general health, and immune-deficiencies caused by certain drugs and diseases such as AIDS make the body vulnerable to certain types of cancer.

Chapter 4

Risk Factors

A risk factor is anything that increases a person's odds of developing a disease such as cancer. Being a woman and growing older are the two most significant risk factors for breast cancer. Because several other experiences and environmental factors seem to be relatively common among women who have the disease, scientists who analyze the incidence of breast cancer have labeled them risk factors. About one-fourth of the women who have breast cancer have only one of the several known risk factors: they are female. And, *risk* is not the same as *cause*. Some women may have several risk factors but never develop the disease.

Because more than one factor is probably involved in triggering a single case of cancer, the disease is often called a multifactorial process. To pinpoint the factors that are most significant, scientists continue to search for some of the biological characteristics, behaviors, and other experiences that women with breast cancer have in common. Once identified, the causes might be avoided, and researchers hope that breast cancer will one day be a preventable disease. Thus far, research cannot identify a single cause—not even the presence of a mutated BRCA 1 or BRCA 2 gene—that always and inevitably leads to cancer. (The gene is named BRCA for "*br*east *ca*ncer.")

There are two main kinds of breast cancer risk factors: (1) inherited risk factors, and (2) lifestyle risk factors, which are external influences such as reproductive history, diet, exercise, and alcohol use. Environmental risk factors such as exposure to chemical pollution or high levels of radiation are important causes of certain types of cancers, but are not thought to be a major cause of breast cancer.

All risk factors are not of equal weight. Certain situations and conditions can put a woman at high risk. For example, if your mother and sister have breast cancer, and you have inherited a mutated BRCA 1 or BRCA 2 gene, you are at a much greater risk of developing the disease than a woman who has no breast cancer in her family. In contrast, women currently using oral contraceptive pills have slightly higher breast cancer risk than women who do not, but this risk is much less than that of women with genetic risk factors. A person who is at high risk for breast cancer for any reason—whether because of her family history or because she has had breast cancer before—needs to discuss with her physician how frequently she should have a clinical breast examination and mammogram, and whether other tests might be helpful.

INHERITED RISK FACTORS

There are two types of hereditary breast cancer: (1) true genetic breast cancer, which accounts for only about 5 to 10 percent of breast cancers, and (2) familial breast cancer, which is more common, accounting for 15 to 20 percent of breast cancers.

Genetic Breast Cancer

Despite the headlines and the debates about genetic testing for breast cancer, only about 5 to 10 percent of breast cancers seem to be caused by an inherited genetic mutation. To develop genetic breast cancer, a woman must inherit a mutated BRCA 1 or BRCA 2 gene—and about one woman in two hundred do. Jewish women of Eastern European descent are at high risk of inheriting the gene: about one in forty of them do. About 50 to 60 percent of women with the mutated form of one of these genes will develop breast cancer by the time they are age seventy. Genetic breast cancer typically affects three or more generations of women in a family. Compared with *sporadic* (not genetic) breast cancer, the genetic type is more likely to occur at a young age and to occur in both breasts.

The first breast cancer gene was identified less than five years ago, so we can expect that other genes linked to breast cancer may be discovered in the near future.

Genetic Errors

One factor contributing to breast cancer, as well as to other types of cancer, appears to be mutations of *tumor suppressor genes* and *oncogenes*. Normally, these genes help cells divide, grow, and die on schedule. Tumor suppressor genes are like a car's brakes, and oncogenes are like the gas pedal. Mutations in tumor suppressor genes inactivate the "brakes" so cells can't stop growing. These mutations may be inherited, but they are usually acquired after birth. Some result from exposure to radiation or cancer-causing chemicals but in most cases no external influence is apparent. Many mutations are thought to occur as random errors in the process that copies a cell's DNA each time it divides. Mutations in oncogenes push the "gas pedal" to the floor and activate the processes involved in cell proliferation.

Researchers have found that inherited mutations of the BRCA 1 or BRCA 2 tumor suppressor genes are responsible for 5 to 10 percent of breast cancers. Inherited mutations of the p53 tumor suppressor genes cause less than 1 percent of breast cancer. But acquired changes in the gene is an important factor in sporadic (not inherited) breast cancers. Acquired mutations of oncogenes, which are involved in the transformation of normal breast cells into cancer, have also been discovered.

The mystery of what causes cancer is beginning to unravel, but identifying all the genes that are involved, as well as learning what can damage them, is an enormous scientific endeavor.

Familial Breast Cancer

Familial breast cancer refers to a tendency among family members to develop this cancer. This tendency may stem from an inherited sensitivity to a particular carcinogen or to radiation. Many experts believe that the majority of cancers are the result of both an inherited susceptibility—though not determined by one particular gene—and one or more lifestyle or environmental factors. Having a family history of cancer increases the risk somewhat, but not to the 50:50 lifetime risk level of someone with the so-called breast cancer gene.

Studies have shown that a woman has a very slightly increased risk even if a third-degree relative, such as a cousin or great-grandmother, has breast cancer. The most significant risk occurs when the family member with cancer is a first-degree relative—mother, sister, or daughter. The risk then increases to three times the usual risk, depending on the woman's age. (The risk is the same if the first-degree relative with breast cancer is a father, brother, or son.)

What does this increased risk actually mean? Suppose your chance of developing breast cancer is 2 in 100 in the next five years. Having a first-degree relative with cancer doubles the risk to 4 in 100 in the same time period. If two first-degree relatives—

a mother and a sister, or two sisters—have the disease, the risk increases to 6 in 100. However, your chance of developing breast cancer rises again if the cancer occurred early in your family member's life or was present in both her breasts. A woman with a relative who developed breast cancer at a young age has a risk two to five times greater than a woman with no close relative with breast cancer.

WHICH BREAST PROBLEMS INCREASE YOUR RISK?

Fluid-filled cysts are very common. They may appear suddenly or grow gradually, and they are sometimes painful. The treatment and the diagnostic test are the same: the doctor inserts a needle into the "lump" and withdraws fluid from it. Ninety-nine percent of the time, an examination of the fluid reveals that the cyst is benign. A history of cysts *does not* increase your risk of breast cancer.

Overproduction of breast epithelial cells has two classifications. In *usual hyperplasia,* the extra cells appear normal under the microscope, and breast cancer risk is slightly increased (by 50 to 100 percent). In *atypical hyperplasia,* the overproduction of abnormal cells increases breast cancer risk by 400 to 500 percent. In other words, the woman is 4 to 5 times more likely to develop breast cancer than are women without this condition.

If you have had a lumpectomy for carcinoma in situ or have had invasive breast cancer, your risk of developing a new cancer, in the same breast or in the opposite breast, increases by 0.5 to 1 percent each year of your life. That means, for example, your risk will be 10 percent higher a decade from now. The condition known as *lobular carcinoma in situ* (LCIS) puts you at the same risk. Although LCIS is an accumulation of abnormal cells within the lobules and not a true cancer, it is a high-risk condition.

LIFESTYLE RISK FACTORS

Reproductive History

One of the most significant biological factors affecting your risk of cancer is your reproductive history—when you began menstruating (*menarche*), when you became pregnant for the first time, and how old you were when you stopped menstruating (*menopause*). All of these events affect the point in time and the length of time your breast cells have been exposed to the female hormones estrogen and progesterone. Exactly how these hormones are involved in breast cancer is still not entirely clear, but they appear to have an important role because breast cancer is so much more common in women than in men.

Many of the changes that occur in breast cell growth and development throughout a woman's life are stimulated by hormones. Some researchers believe that estrogen influences premalignant cells in the breast, causing them to become malignant. Another theory is that there are phases in a woman's life when the balance between estrogen and progesterone is slightly off, such as at menarche and again at menopause. During these times, some scientists speculate, estrogen may be carcinogenic. Another explanation is that when the breast is still in a nonfunctioning state—that is, from the time menstruation begins until the first pregnancy—the breast cells are more sensitive to cancer-causing agents in the environment.

Women who have many menstrual cycles during their lives—those who have early (before twelve) menarche and/or late menopause (after fifty-five), and never have children—seem to be more likely to develop breast cancer than women who do not experience as many menstrual cycles. Women who have children at a young age (before about thirty) seem to be at lower risk than women who have children later in life.

Pregnancy does seem to be protective of the breasts. In addition to disrupting the menstrual cycle and altering the balance of female hormones, pregnancy allows the breast cells to develop fully and prepare to produce milk, possibly making the cells less susceptible to cancer-causing influences. However, this benefit of pregnancy is significant only if a woman has her first child before age thirty.

Only a slight increase in risk is associated with taking estrogen replacement therapy (ERT) or hormone replacement therapy (HRT) after menopause. A moderate risk (about a 35 percent increase) has been reported for those taking ERT for a prolonged time, such as ten years.

When women who have used ERT discontinue the treatment, their risk returns to normal in about five years. However, ERT lowers a woman's risk of heart disease, osteoporosis, and some other conditions, and these factors must be weighed by a woman and her physician.

At one time, researchers suspected that a miscarriage increased a woman's risk of breast cancer, and several studies suggested that induced (intentional) abortion increased the risk. Recently, however, a large study conducted in Denmark showed that women who had induced abortions had no increased risk for breast cancer even after long follow-up.

A controversial issue has been whether taking birth control pills (both the low-dose pills common today and the high-estrogen pills that were common when oral contraceptives were first introduced) puts a woman at risk for breast cancer. A 1996 study analyzed data from more than twenty international sources and found a slightly increased risk in women taking oral contraceptives but no excess risk ten or more years after quitting "the pill." Breast cancers diagnosed in current or previous oral contraceptive users have tended to be less advanced than those in nonusers. These two effects (more cases and less spread at the time of diagnosis) may balance each other out to some degree. Experts are still not sure whether oral contraceptives increase, decrease, or have no effect on a woman's risk of dying of breast cancer.

Location

Scientists believe that some factors in the environment are involved in the development of breast cancer: (1) because the incidence of breast cancer varies geographically, and (2) because when people migrate from one location to another, the risk of developing specific cancers shifts, particularly among the second generation of people in the new locale. Research has also revealed that the way people live—lifestyle factors such as what they eat and drink, and how much they exercise—may have an impact on their risk of developing cancer. Because people living in different areas eat different foods, regional diet and other lifestyle factors may be important in explaining geographical variations in cancer risk. Scientists are continuing to take a close look at factors ranging from diet to pollution.

Diet

It has long been surmised that fat in the diet is linked to the development of breast cancer. People who live in parts of the world where there is little fat in the diet have a lower risk than those who live where higher quantities of dietary fat are common. Furthermore, when people who live where the incidence of breast cancer is low—most notably, the Japanese—move to areas where a high-fat diet is the norm, their incidence of the disease increases, and the risk among their children, the second generation of residents, is even higher. Although differences in dietary fat content help to explain why breast cancer rates differ around the world, there is no conclusive evidence that Americans with high- and low-fat diets have different levels of breast cancer risk.

A high-fat diet also increases the likelihood of obesity. Fat cells are known to produce estrogens, which may affect the breast cells, but researchers also point out that increased body fat raises insulin levels, which may also stimulate tumor growth. In one study of more than 1,500 women, researchers discovered that those in their fifties who had recently gained more than ten pounds had three times the risk of developing breast cancer, compared to those with no weight change. The connection between body weight and breast cancer risk is complex. Many other factors, such as hormone replacement therapy, or whether a woman gained weight early or late in life, my be relevant.

Exercise

Hormonal effects may also explain why women who lead active lives are at lower risk of developing breast cancer than sedentary women. Recently, a study of more than 25,000 pre- and post-menopausal women revealed that those who exercised during their leisure time had a 37 percent lower risk of breast cancer than their inactive counterparts, and women whose jobs involved physical exertion had an even greater risk reduction. Earlier studies had shown that regular exercise can protect against several types of cancer, but this new research indicates that the American Cancer Society's recommendation to be at least moderately active for thirty minutes on most days of the week is especially important in preventing breast cancer.

Alcohol

In several large studies, drinking alcohol has been consistently associated with an increased risk of breast cancer, as well as mouth, throat, esophageal, and liver cancer. A drink a day may increase the risk by as much as 40 percent. According to one study, drinking before age thirty poses an even greater risk than drinking later in life. For this reason, the American Cancer Society recommends limiting consumption of alcohol at all ages, or not drinking at all.

Pollution/Pesticides

Whether environmental pollutants and pesticides cause breast cancer has been hotly debated for decades. Because DDE,* a metabolite of the insecticide DDT, accumulates in fatty tissue of the breast and can remain there for a long time, people wondered whether the pesticide played a role in breast cancer development. Indeed, a small study some years ago suggested that there was a link. Recently, however, a study of more than 120,000 women found that there was no correlation between DDE or PCB levels in women and breast cancer. The federal government banned use of both DDT and PCBs in the United States years ago, but they persist in the environment.

Prevention

Many factors that put women at risk, such as family history and gender, are obviously beyond their control. But women can improve their bodies' defenses against breast cancer. In 1996, the American Cancer Society updated its "Guidelines on Diet, Nutrition, and Cancer Prevention" (see page 51) to incorporate the most recent research on reducing the risk of all types of cancer. Studies suggest that about one-third of the 500,000 cancer

* DDE = dichlordiphenylethylene.

deaths that occur each year are from cancers whose cause is related to diet. Physical activity has also proved to be an important factor. And, of course, quitting smoking is essential to prevent a variety of cancers, although no specific link to breast cancer has been established.

AMERICAN CANCER SOCIETY GUIDELINES ON DIET, NUTRITION, AND CANCER PREVENTION

1. Choose most of the foods you eat from plant sources:
   - Eat five or more servings of fruits and vegetables each day.
   - Eat breads, cereals, grain products, rice, pasta, or beans several times a day.
2. Limit your intake of high-fat foods, particularly those from animal sources:
   - Choose foods low in fat.
   - Limit consumption of meats, especially high-fat meats.
3. Be physically active; achieve and maintain a healthy weight:
   - Be at least moderately active for thirty minutes or more on most days of the week.
   - Stay within your healthy weight range.
4. Limit your consumption of alcoholic beverages, if you drink at all.

Chapter 5

Diagnosis

When breast cancer is detected early—that is, when it is still confined to the breast and has not spread to the lymph nodes—the five-year survival rate is 97 percent. Despite this encouraging fact, there's no question that discovering a lump in your breast, or hearing your physician tell you that something about your breast feels suspicious, or having a questionable area appear on your mammogram is frightening. You may want to think, "Oh, it's nothing," and dismiss it, but you must be smart and have the breast evaluated. This prediagnostic phase is focused on having the appropriate examinations and tests. Sometimes, the possibility of breast cancer is ruled out early in the test process. If it isn't, the order of events is usually to:

1. See your doctor for a clinical breast exam.
2. See a breast specialist for a clinical breast exam.
3. Have a diagnostic mammogram and, in some cases, diagnostic ultrasound imaging.
4. Have a biopsy.

Depending on how the abnormality is discovered, and by whom, these steps, or their sequence, may vary.

There are so many fears . . . so many emotions that come up. There are just so many thoughts of: What's going to happen to me? Am I going to be dead next year? What is the outcome going to be? For me, the hardest thing to deal with is the range of fears and anxiety. I've tried to deal with it with meditation, visualization, and having conversations with people about it.

—J.C.

WHAT YOUR DOCTOR WILL DO

Typically, the first step if you discover a lump is to see your doctor. He or she will perform a clinical breast exam (see Chapter 2), ask you to have a diagnostic mammogram, and, regardless of the results of that X-ray, may refer you to a breast surgeon. The surgeon will also palpate your breasts and underarm areas and may order additional tests, such as ultrasound imaging. Depending on the results of the breast exams and other tests, a biopsy is the next and final diagnostic step.

During all this activity, you have two main jobs: (1) make *and keep* the necessary appointments without delay, and (2) try not to panic. Some women are so fearful of cancer that they postpone calling their doctor when they feel something unusual in their breast. Others are so terrified that nothing short of an ambulance can get them to the doctor soon enough. Although an emergency visit is not necessary, when you call your doctor's office, indicate that there is some urgency. You'll have fewer sleepless nights spent worrying.

The days of waiting to see different doctors and receive test results are difficult and uncertain. Enlist all the resources and

THE CRITICAL FIRST STEP: CALLING YOUR DOCTOR

Most women discover breast abnormalities themselves, accidentally or by doing BSE. But the fact is that breast cancer can be difficult to diagnose and its progress is hard to predict. Even a mammogram is not foolproof. Mammograms may give false-negative results: A lump that is malignant, for example, may not appear on the breast X-ray at all. Similarly, a lump discovered during a clinical breast exam can be misdiagnosed. A lump that feels like a cyst may be a solid tumor, and some solid, smooth tumors turn out to be breast cancer and not the benign masses they appear to be. A physician will usually do a biopsy to rule out even the smallest chance of a malignancy. Having a biopsy on tissue that turns out to be benign is better than not having one and missing the key early-stage detection of breast cancer.

A more difficult issue is the questionable lump. The area may be normal, but when the results of a physical examination of the breasts are inconclusive, a follow-up exam may be very important. In premenopausal women, this may be as soon as one week after the next menstrual period. In postmenopausal women, a follow up in two to four months is more usual.

activities you rely on to deal with the stresses of your life—talking with a close friend, taking long walks, going to the movies, or practicing relaxation exercises. Having a friend or family member accompany you to the various appointments can provide both distraction and support.

FINDING A BREAST SURGEON

If your gynecologist or family physician detects something abnormal during a breast exam, or there is a suspicious area on your mammogram, ask for a referral to a breast specialist—a board-certified surgeon who is an expert in oncology or cancer surgery and who also specializes in breast problems. If your gynecologist or family doctor cannot recommend someone, call one of the Comprehensive Cancer Centers recognized by the National Cancer Institute (see the Resources section that follows Chapter 21). It's important to seek one or more expert opinions as soon as you can. You will then feel confident that you have done everything possible to obtain an accurate diagnosis.

BREAST CANCER DETECTION

Chances are high that if you are premenopausal, a lump you discover while examining your breasts is not cancer. If you've gone through menopause, those same chances are about 50:50. And if you're over age seventy, there is greater risk that the lump you feel is malignant. No matter what your age or your risk, the only way to be sure that a lump or a suspicious area is not cancer is to have appropriate diagnostic tests done promptly.

In the past, "tests" for breast cancer meant only one thing: a *biopsy*, which is the removal of tissue for microscopic examination. Today, however, other preliminary tests can help determine whether a biopsy is necessary. Nevertheless, the only way to definitively diagnose—or rule out—breast cancer is with a biopsy.

DIAGNOSTIC MAMMOGRAPHY

A diagnostic mammogram is similar to a screening mammogram (see Chapter 2) except that it may involve more than two views of each breast, and views from different angles. Your doctor may refer you to a radiologist for this test: (1) if something abnormal has been detected on a screening mammogram, (2) if anything out of the ordinary is noticed during a clinical breast examination, or (3) if you have a nipple discharge. A diagnostic mammogram is sometimes recommended for women with breast implants if the radiologist doesn't believe the usual screening mammogram will reveal all the breast tissue.

Because they understand your anxiety regarding the results of a diagnostic mammogram, most radiologists will review the images immediately following the X-ray and will let you know, within a few minutes, whether any abnormality is noted at first glance. A more careful reading will follow, and a report will be sent to your physician.

Many breast conditions create a distinct white image on the X-ray. A benign, fluid-filled cyst, or a benign, fibrous, and glandular tumor (a *fibroadenoma*) is usually round and self-contained; a malignant tumor typically has a rough surface and fibers can be seen extending from it. But some conditions—a scar or an area of tissue damaged by injury (*fat necrosis*)—can actually pull on surrounding tissue and create a pucker like lesion, just as cancer does. Sometimes, particularly in younger women, the breast tissue is very dense and it may be impossible to see a lesion within it. The radiologist will note this on the report in medical terms that may sound like a disease. When you review the report with your doctor, ask for an explanation of any terminology that you don't understand. Clusters of so-called *microcalcifications*, for instance, are tiny white spots that indicate cancer about 18 percent to 25 percent of the time.

Reading mammograms is not an exact science, and even radiologists who specialize in analyzing breast X-rays can disagree when they interpret what they see. Therefore, it's perfectly acceptable to ask for a second opinion from another radiologist, preferably one who specializes in diagnosing breast cancer. Ask your gynecologist or family physician for a recommendation, and/or locate a breast cancer center associated with a major teaching institution in your area. You probably will not need to have another mammogram. You can take the earlier X-ray film to the consulting radiologist, or have it sent, but be prepared for a request to get a different view of the breast.

Depending on what appears on your mammogram, the radiologist and/or your physician may suggest that you return in six months for a repeat X-ray. This is especially likely when you have your first mammogram, because no previous X-ray is available for comparison. If the spot under consideration is drawing only a low level of suspicion, then experience and judgment are required to make a good recommendation. A second opinion can be a good idea.

One criticism of mammography is that, with improved technology, many benign tissue formations that may not have even appeared on earlier mammographic X-rays are now obvious. And, because some women are so frightened, and their physicians certainly don't want to ignore a potentially malignant lesion, more biopsies are being done on benign conditions. In such cases, the mammogram report is a false-positive one.

DIAGNOSTIC ULTRASOUND

Ultrasonography involves using short bursts or pulses of high-frequency sound waves to create an image. The pattern of echoes that occurs as the pulses of sound bounce off the breast tissue is altered by any abnormal areas, such as a cyst or a solid mass. The echo pattern is converted by a computer into visible points on a video display terminal and recorded so that a doctor can review them and make still images for closer study.

Ultrasound can be used on various parts of the body to detect tumors. On the breast, a handheld device that emits sound waves, called a transducer, is rubbed firmly over the skin. A special jelly is applied first, so that the transducer glides over the breast easily and smoothly, and the sound waves penetrate without interruption. The test is not painful. There is pressure as the breast is compressed, but not as much as with a mammogram. Depending on the clarity of the image and the breast size, among other factors, ultrasonography takes from a few minutes to just under half an hour.

The image created with ultrasound cannot convey whether a tumor is malignant; rather, it is used primarily to distinguish between fluid-filled cysts, which are virtually always benign, and solid tumors, which may require a biopsy. As in a mammogram, a cyst typically appears smooth and round. Few, if any, "echos" or irregular sound waves are found in an ultrasound image of a cyst, whereas cancer has irregular borders. Even though ultrasonography can be useful in specific instances, it is generally not accurate enough to be used as a screening test for breast cancer. The test is sometimes done: (1) if a woman or her doctor feels something unusual but the mammogram is negative; (2) if a woman has very dense breasts that cannot be visualized very well by mammography; or (3) if a woman has breast implants. Occasionally, ultrasonography is used to locate a tumor and guide the physician's placement of a needle to aspirate fluid or retrieve a tissue sample.

BIOPSY

Examining cells under a microscope is the only way to determine whether they are malignant. (This exam is done by a *pathologist*, a physician who specializes in recognizing microscopic abnormalities of cells and tissues.) Depending on the type of biopsy done and the results of the laboratory analysis, sampling the tissue a second time is occasionally necessary. Learning that you need to have a biopsy is a frightening experience, so it should help to know that only two out of ten breast lumps examined microscopically are malignant.

Tissue can be removed from the breast in a variety of ways. The critical objective is to get enough tissue from the right area. By using mammography or ultrasonography to assist the procedure, clusters of cells that haven't yet formed a detectable lump can be precisely sampled (see the section on stereotactic biopsy, on pages 62–63).

In the past, if it was suspected that a lump was malignant, a surgeon would perform what is called a *one-step procedure*. In this method, the woman received general anesthesia and a sample of tissue was retrieved and immediately examined by a pathologist. If it was malignant, a mastectomy was done. Fifteen or twenty years ago, it wasn't unusual for a woman to go to an operating room for a biopsy and wake up to find her breast had been removed. Today, surgeons recognize that the time between diagnosis and surgical treatment is not as crucial as was once thought, and that there are other treatments besides a mastectomy.

In a *two-step procedure*, the diagnostic test—the biopsy—is done at one time and, if it is positive for cancer, the lump or the breast is removed later, in a separate surgery. This allows a woman time to gather information, discuss treatment options with her family or significant other, and seek a second or even a third opinion.

Fine-Needle Aspiration Biopsy (FNAB)

The quickest, simplest, least expensive, least uncomfortable, and least traumatic way to sample breast tissue is to have a physician

---

INFORMED CONSENT

Before undergoing a surgical biopsy, you will be asked to sign an informed consent document, confirming that you've been told the reasons for the biopsy, the kind of biopsy that will be done, and any potential side effects or complications that might result. (Needle procedures may not require a formal signed consent.) In rare instances, a woman may choose to have a one-step procedure if cancer is found. The consent document will then state that the surgeon has permission to perform a mastectomy under the same anesthesia.

---

with experience in doing breast biopsy do a fine-needle aspiration biopsy (FNAB). You may hear the procedure called by several combinations of these terms—fine-needle biopsy, aspiration biopsy, or fine-needle aspiration—or referred to as suction biopsy. A needle even smaller than the one used to withdraw blood is attached to a hypodermic syringe. The physician cleanses the skin with an antiseptic and then holds the lump securely with one hand. With the opposite hand, he or she inserts the needle through the skin and into the lump. By moving the needle slightly back and forth and pulling back on the hypodermic, a tiny bit of tissue or fluid is retrieved. There is a little discomfort, but it lasts only a few seconds. Then the sample is placed on a glass slide for a microscopic examination.

When a suspicious lesion is small and cannot be felt on physical examination, a needle biopsy may be done while the radiologist or surgeon views the breast on a mammogram (see the section on stereotactic biopsy, on pages 62–63).

If the lump turns out to be a fluid-filled, benign cyst, the fluid is withdrawn and the walls of the cyst collapse. For 99 percent of cysts, that is the only procedure needed. If the fluid is blood-tinged or otherwise abnormal, a pathologist may examine a sample of the fluid, searching for cancer cells.

The main requirement for FNAB is that a doctor skilled in performing this type of biopsy must be able to feel the lump clearly, or, alternatively, must have experience in ultrasound-guided or stereotactic needle biopsy, in order to target the needle correctly.

There are situations in which FNAB must be followed by another kind of biopsy or by surgery. For example, when the biopsy shows no cancer cells but the abnormality still appears on the mammogram, or when the doctor feels a suspicious mass, another procedure may be needed. Some physicians consider fine-needle aspiration biopsy to be one in a series of three tests, along with clinical breast examination and mammography. If the FNAB is negative and the other two tests are positive, another type of biopsy is necessary. When the FNAB is negative, the sample may have been insufficient, or the needle may have missed its target and withdrawn only nearby benign cells.

Core Needle Biopsy

If a fine-needle aspiration biopsy fails to confirm a diagnosis, or a larger tissue sample is required, a core needle biopsy may be the next step. The breast surgeon removes a "core" of tissue by using a hollow needle about the size of a ball point pen refill, with a cutting edge. It is pushed into the anesthetized breast tissue from a special biopsy gun. Then the needle—containing a tiny cylinder of tissue about an inch long—is withdrawn. Sometimes, the surgeon repeats the process to retrieve multiple samples. Although a local anesthetic is used, the procedure still causes the pain of needle puncture, which varies according to how close to the nipple the biopsy needle is and how dense the tissue is. A single stitch may be necessary to suture closed the hole made by the core needle. Core needle biopsy may also be done using the stereotactic method (see below) or in conjunction with ultrasound.

Stereotactic Biopsy

Stereotactic biopsy is a core biopsy or, less often, an FNAB of a nonpalpable lump. A computer scans "stereo" mammogram images to create a three-dimensional image of the breast. Then the computer aims the core biopsy gun at the precise location of an abnormal lesion. Before the automated gun is "fired," the skin over the breast is cleaned with an antiseptic, a local anesthetic is injected, and a tiny incision is made where the needle will enter the breast. Several biopsies can be done in a few minutes. This method is especially useful for lesions that are too small to be felt but can be seen on a mammogram.

As automated stereotactic biopsy equipment becomes more widely available, fewer surgical biopsies (see "Open Biopsy," on pages 63–65) will be necessary. The techniques are nearly equal in their 90 to 95 percent accuracy rates. The method is also less expensive than surgery, and some experts predict that it will become the standard method for sampling nonpalpable lesions detected by mammography.

In 1997, a new stereotactic device called Mammotome became available. It uses a probe to retrieve the breast tissue and, because the probe has a side opening and a high-speed rotating cutter within, it can be turned to allow suction to pull tissue into the "window" on the side of the probe. In this way, several biopsies can be obtained with only one insertion of the probe, and the tissue samples removed are larger than those obtained with a core biopsy needle. This probe device may be safer in retrieving biopsies from women with breast implants, which could leak if punctured with a biopsy needle.

Open Biopsy

To perform an open or surgical biopsy, the surgeon makes an incision in the anesthetized breast. There are two situations in which surgery is done after a needle biopsy: (1) when the pathologist cannot determine whether the tissue retrieved with a needle biopsy is malignant, and (2) when the surgeon needs to confirm the findings of a fine- or core-needle biopsy. (If the mammogram or clinical breast exam indicates clearly that a lump should be removed, the surgeon will proceed directly to open biopsy, regardless of its nature on FNA.) A surgical biopsy can be an *excisional biopsy*, in which the entire lump is removed, or an *incisional biopsy*, in which a part of the lump or abnormal area is removed.

If it is difficult for the surgeon to locate the lump, or if the abnormality is very small, a very fine wire may be placed into the lesion, while the surgeon or a radiologist views the placement of the wire on a mammogram. The wire is then left in place, marking the tissue that is to be immediately sampled for a surgical biopsy. This procedure is called *wire localization*.

If you are treated in a surgery center or hospital, it is not necessary to stay overnight, but be prepared to spend the day in the surgery center. You will have some blood tests, and your temperature, blood pressure, and pulse rate will be recorded. If you have monitored sedation or general anesthesia, you will not be able to eat or drink after midnight prior to surgery. The procedure is done in an operating suite.

An incisional biopsy is almost always done under local anesthesia. The incision is smaller than that needed for an excisional biopsy, because the surgeon is removing only a tiny wedge of the lump or area. A local anesthetic can be used for an excisional biopsy, but if it is done in a free-standing or ambulatory surgery center, monitored sedation or general anesthesia can be used. Only rarely is general anesthesia needed.

For an *excisional* biopsy, after the skin is cleansed and anesthetized with a local anesthetic, an incision is made in the breast, and the mass, along with a *margin* of tissue around it, is *excised*, or removed. (In some cases, this is the equivalent of a lumpectomy [see Chapter 7], and no further removal of breast tissue is required.)

Analysis of the tumor and the tissue margin may begin in the laboratory while you are still in the operating room. The pathologist quick-freezes a portion of the tissue. Thin slices of the frozen sample are put on slides and stained with dyes that make the tissue easier to see under a microscope. The freezing process distorts the tissue somewhat, and these frozen sections will not provide as comprehensive and detailed a picture as the *permanent sections*, which are made from the tissue at a later time. If the tissue is small or difficult to handle, it may not be appropriate for the pathologist to prepare a frozen section. The frozen section takes about ten to twenty minutes. In the days of the one-step procedure, the frozen section was an important guide for the surgeon. Now, it may be done to give an immediate answer to the woman. But because freezing may distort the tissue, some surgeons choose not to use this method at all, particularly if the tumor is small.

To prepare a permanent section, a laboratory technician embeds a sample of tissue in a special wax. Slices made from this block are placed on a slide, stained, and viewed under a microscope by a pathologist. The details of the tissue and its cells are more distinct on a permanent section than on a frozen section. This process generally takes one to two days, but may take longer if extra slices of the tissue are needed to make an accurate diagnosis.

When the lump or suspicious area has been removed, the surgeon closes the wound with a few stitches. Then you are moved to the recovery room. If a frozen section was done, then, by the time you are awake, the surgeon may be able to give you the most important result of your biopsy—whether it showed breast cancer or a benign condition. If the lump is malignant, removing it may be the only treatment to the breast that is necessary, depending on the size of the tumor and provided the margin of tissue around the cancer shows no signs of malignancy. If there are cancer cells in the removed tissue at the margin, another operation is usually necessary, although a small amount of cancer remaining at one edge may be treated by increasing the radiation dose (see Chapter 7).

Chapter 6

If the Diagnosis Is Cancer

After a diagnosis is made, you will meet with your doctor to review the results of your biopsy and begin discussing treatment options. Women are sometimes surprised to learn that treatment decisions may not yet be clear-cut. Surgery is needed if the entire lump was not removed at the time the biopsy was done. The tissue sample may require some additional very specific testing, or, sometimes, lymph nodes that were not removed during the initial surgery may now be taken out for examination. If surgery has been done, this is also the time when your cancer is staged (see pages 76–80). Also, this is the time to get a second opinion from another breast surgeon and possibly another pathologist. This diagnostic phase consists of three essential steps:

1. Discuss the biopsy report with your breast surgeon. You may also want to speak with the pathologist who examined the specimen.
2. Seek a second opinion.
3. Understand the stage of your cancer (if surgery has been done and has revealed a malignancy).

TAKING ACTION

By this time, you may be weary of being prodded, poked, and tested, but a few additional examinations are important. When you get a second opinion, the new physician will probably do a clinical breast examination, and you may need to have another mammogram of one or both breasts.

When cancer is diagnosed by a fine needle aspiration biopsy, a core biopsy, or an incisional biopsy, the doctor will want to schedule surgery to remove the entire lump promptly. In some cases, this is all the treatment that will be necessary (see Chapter 7). In other cases, the surgeon will remove the lump, and then determine whether a mastectomy (removal of the breast) and/or underarm lymph nodes is necessary. To prepare for surgery, you may have urine and blood tests and possibly a chest X-ray and electrocardiogram.

During this first postbiopsy meeting, your doctor will tell you, in detail, what the pathologist found when examining your breast tissue. More information will be forthcoming when the entire lump is removed.

BRING A FRIEND WITH YOU

You should bring someone along on this visit, for support and for help in sorting and remembering the information given to you. Later, when you're trying to recollect what was said and review what you've learned, your friend or family member can jog your memory and offer feedback. Some physicians give permission to tape-record the consultation, because they understand that you are under a great deal of stress and may have difficulty remembering certain details of the discussion. At the very least,

My husband has been so supportive since the beginning. He really took over. When I came home and told him the diagnosis, he was, of course, upset and crying. But then he said, "I'm going to start making phone calls." He's been in the medical field as a salesman for almost twenty years, so he knew people to call. My husband and I really take charge of our health care, because you have to.

—P.S.

bring a notebook and pen, so you can take notes on what your doctor tells you.

One study has shown that the way we interpret what we hear is affected by many things, including our family history. If you lost a mother or sister to breast cancer, your interpretation of the facts about your own cancer will be very different from that of a woman whose mother or sister is a longtime survivor of the disease. Having someone else present when your doctor gives you diagnostic information is helpful because you may be uncertain of what the diagnosis means or you may want to talk it over with someone who was also listening.

SECOND OPINION

There are no hard and fast rules for what type of biopsy and/or surgery is done for which type and size of suspected cancer, but there are general guidelines. Your doctor will individualize the diagnostic process and make treatment recommendations based on your needs. Understand, though, that the surgeon's own experience is a factor in this equation. And be aware that doctors are influenced by the resources and protocols of the facility where they work. That is why getting a second or even a third opinion from a breast specialist at another medical center, *before* you make your final treatment decision, is so important.

Any uncertainty about the diagnosis or the type and aggressiveness of the cancer cells may prompt your physician to get a second pathology opinion. This is also something you can seek for yourself; ask your breast specialist to recommend a pathologist. Or, if you are planning to see another breast specialist for a second opinion, you may want to bring your pathology slides with you. The second breast specialist can have another pathologist look at the slides and perhaps do additional tests.

DESCRIBING *YOUR* CANCER

Not all breast cancers are alike. Some are very slow to develop and grow; others progress quite rapidly. When a surgical biopsy or lumpectomy is done and the microscopic examination confirms that cancer cells are present, the doctor's next step is to analyze *prognostic factors*—characteristics that reveal how aggressive the malignant cells are. Some of these prognostic factors can be determined early, based on tissue obtained from a needle or core biopsy, but others require testing of larger tissue samples, which cannot be done until the entire cancer is removed. The pathologist's analysis that follows discusses these specific tests. Consequently, treatment options may be modified according to these prognostic factors.

Cancer under the Microscope

The pathologist first determines whether the cells are malignant. When cancer is present, the pathologist identifies the type of cancer, the size of the tumor, and its grade (see pages 72–74). The cancer cells themselves are examined, and if a margin of tissue

CARCINOMA IN SITU

Now that mammography is in widespread use, more breast cancer is being diagnosed at its very earliest stage—*carcinoma in situ*. When abnormal cells are confined to the lobules without invading the surrounding tissue, it is called *lobular carcinoma in situ* or *lobular neoplasia*. When the abnormal cells are confined to the ducts, the diagnosis is *ductal carcinoma in situ*.

Lobular Carcinoma in Situ (LCIS)
LCIS is not considered a true cancer because it is believed that these cells do not actually become cancer even if they are not removed. However, LCIS is considered a risk factor for breast cancer development in either breast in the future.

Unlike DCIS (see below), LCIS does not usually appear on a mammogram but is diagnosed only when a biopsy is taken for some other reason. After the diagnosis of LCIS, the risk of breast cancer development is only about 1 percent per year for about fifteen years.

Ductal Carcinoma in Situ (DCIS)
In contrast, DCIS does have the potential to eventually become invasive although the process may take several years.

A DCIS is usually too small to feel but tends to be diagnosed when calcium deposits *(microcalcifications)* form in clusters of abnormal cells and appear on a mammogram.

There is currently a great deal of controversy about the treatment of DCIS. A series of clinical trials is under way to discover ways to determine which cases of DCIS are more aggressive and under what circumstances more or less treatment is needed.

Research is currently under way to determine whether hormone therapy, such as tamoxifen, will prevent recurrences of intraductal cancer. If it does, the drug may become standard treatment for this condition.

In one survey of about 20,000 cases of DCIS across the country, 75 percent of women had mastectomies. Critics argue that many of these operations were unnecessary because, for many of the women, the lesions may not have become invasive for years, if at all. Further-more, many could have been effectively treated by breast conserva-tion. Use of this surgery for DCIS has been declining: Between 1983 and 1992, there were 27 percent fewer mastectomies for DCIS. The number treated by lumpectomy with radiation therapy increased about 17 percent, and those treated by lumpectomy alone increased almost 11 percent during those years.

from around a lump has been removed for examination, the pathologist determines whether the cancer extends into that tissue.

THE PATHOLOGY REPORT

All the information about the microscopic examination will be in the pathologist's report. Some reports are brief and quickly sum-marize the findings; others are quite long and involved. In either case, after reviewing the report with your doctor, you may ask for a copy to take home.

In most facilities, a labeled sample of your core or surgical biopsy is stored within small (about half-inch) blocks of wax in the laboratory, so that your doctor can have additional micro-scope slides (called *recuts*) made for other tests that may be needed. You can request slides of your tumor from the laboratory (you may have to pay a fee) if you want a second opinion from an-other pathologist. An FNAB doesn't usually retrieve enough tis-sue to save in wax, but the microscope slides are always available for review by a second specialist.

THE PATHOLOGIST'S ANALYSIS

The absolutely most important predictor of whether the cancer has spread to the rest of the body, or is likely to in the future, is the presence of cancer cells in the lymph nodes near the breast. This is why lymph nodes are usually *sampled*—removed at the time of surgery and examined to see whether they contain cancer cells. Tumor size and tumor grade (see below) are also important interacting predictors. All other cellular tests run far behind these characteristics in terms of determining the cancer's ability to spread. Tests on the tumor cells were designed for their predictive value, and it was hoped that they would help a woman avoid having the lymph nodes under her arm removed. The cellular tests may be helpful in some cases, but, as predictors of cancer's spread, their results are not as accurate as knowing whether lymph nodes are involved and, if so, how many nodes contain cancer cells.

THE CANCER TYPE

Almost all invasive breast cancers are adenocarcinomas (see Chapter 3), and most breast adenocarcinomas (about 80 percent) are *ductal carcinomas*, meaning they arise from the ducts. About 10 percent are *lobular carcinomas*, which start in the lobules. Both types of cancer may spread to the lymph nodes under the arms, which is why lymph nodes are removed and examined for cancer cells (see Chapter 7).

About 10 percent of adenocarcinomas are uncommon types, such as medullary (5 to 7 percent), mucinous (3 percent), and tubular (1 to 3 percent). These tend to indicate a better prognosis than ductal or lobular carcinomas. There are a few other types of breast cancer, such as squamous cell carcinomas, cystosarcoma phyllodes, and angiosarcoma, but these are very rare and are treated differently than the various adenocarcinomas.

Inflammatory breast cancer accounts for about 1 percent of all breast cancers. The name of this disease was chosen many years ago because the breast appears to be inflamed: it is red, feels warm, and swells, and the skin may thicken to the consistency of an orange peel. Although doctors now know that these signs are not due to inflammation, but rather to spread of breast cancer to lymphatic channels in the skin, the name "inflammatory cancer" remains. Unlike the other rare breast cancer types that are diagnosed by the microscopic appearance of their cells, the key feature of inflammatory cancer is its pattern of spread.

THE TUMOR GRADE

One of the pathologist's most important tasks is to try to ascertain how aggressive the cancer is—how likely it is to grow rapidly and spread to other organs. Even a small tumor can be fast-growing and aggressive if it is high-grade. This will appear on the pathology report as *tumor grade*. Various systems have been devised to grade tumors, so you may see classifications or numbers that are different from those that appear in this chapter (pages 76–80). Ask your doctor to spend a few minutes reviewing your pathology report with you and explaining what the terms and numbers mean. Also, because pathologists can differ in their analysis of a tumor's grade, you may want to get more than one opinion.

Nuclear grade is an indication of how closely the nucleus of the cell (the center part of the cell, which contains its DNA) resembles that of normal breast cells. Tumor nuclear grade is rated on a scale of one to three, with grade three predicting the greatest degree of aggressiveness. Instead of giving cancer cells a number grade, the pathologist may simply indicate that a cancer is high-grade (likely to be fast-growing) or low-grade (likely to be slow-growing).

Histologic tumor grade is an indication of the architecture of the cells in relationship to each other, as well as features of individual cells. Grade 1 cancers contain relatively normal-looking cells that do not appear to be growing rapidly and are arranged in small tubules. Grade 3 cancers lack these features and tend to grow and spread more aggressively. Grades 1, 2, and 3 cancers are sometimes called, respectively, well differentiated, moderately differentiated, and poorly differentiated.

Other factors that affect prognosis will be considered when planning your treatment, but knowledge of grade can be important.

YOUR HORMONE RECEPTOR STATUS

Receptors for estrogen on a cancer cell means that the cancer cell can bind with this female hormone. There is another type of protein receptor for the other female hormone, progesterone. The status of progesterone and estrogen receptors can generally predict a woman's response to hormone therapy and, sometimes, the chances that the cancer will recur.

If estrogen receptors (ER) are present, the tumor is said to be ER positive. These cancer cells are usually well differentiated and indicate a better prognosis than if the tumor is ER negative. If progesterone receptors (PR) are present, the tumor is PR positive. Tumors with a high percentage of estrogen receptors are often high in progesterone receptors, and such a combination indicates a cancer will be "easier" to treat—that is, with hormonal manipulation, the outcome is more likely to be favorable.

Today, the estrogen-receptor-blocking drug tamoxifen is frequently prescribed, so learning whether you have hormone receptors is essential (see Chapter 9). The presence and intensity of hormone receptors are related to age, and cancer cells in older women are more likely to have more of them.

Other Tests

Pathologists may use other tests and measures in an attempt to learn which cancers must be treated with high doses of strong drugs, and which ones are so slow-growing that they are unlikely to spread to other parts of the body and thus don't require chemotherapy. Currently, experts are uncertain whether these methods have any consistently accurate and predictive value in and of themselves. But when they are considered along with other tests, your doctor may get a clearer picture of your cancer. Here are a few tests that you may hear about, especially if you are treated in a research institution.

FLOW CYTOMETRY

One indicator of a tumor's aggressiveness relies on a technique called *flow cytometry*, a method of measuring the DNA *index* or *ploidy* of cancer cells (the amount of DNA they contain). If there's a normal amount of DNA, the cells are said to be *diploid*. If the amount if abnormal, the cells are described as *aneuploid*. Flow cytometry can also measure the *S-phase fraction*—the percentage of cells in a sample that are in a particular stage of cell division called the *synthesis* phase. The more cells that are in this S-phase, the faster the tissue is growing, and the more aggressive the cancer is likely to be. Flow cytometry is a test with technical challenges and some sampling error. Laboratories rely on different techniques to perform many of these tests, so comparing results of examinations done by various labs is not always advisable. Only one-thousandth or less of a typical tumor is submitted for this test, and this small fraction may not be representative of the whole. In contrast, nuclear grade and histologic grade can be determined by microscopic examination of the slides that contain multiple slices from several areas of the tumor.

Tests for the Future

Several other characteristics are being analyzed experimentally. They include:

- *HER-2/neu* is an oncogene (see Chapter 3) that is present in larger than normal quantities in about one third of breast cancers. This causes overproduction of a protein that stimulates cell growth, and its presence may indicate that the tumor is more aggressive. A new drug, Herceptin, is now available that specifically disrupts the growth of cancer cells with too much HER-2/neu protein. The HER-2/neu test is useful in predicting which women with breast cancer are likely to benefit from this new treatment.
- *Epidermal growth factor* receptors help regulate cancer cell growth. When there is an increase in their number, it may indicate the tumor is fast-growing.
- *Angiogenesis* is the formation of small blood vessels, and breast cancer cells can secrete substances that promote the growth of these vessels. They help nourish the tumor and promote a pathway for metastasis. There are methods for counting the number of vessels around the edge of a tumor, which will reflect how aggressive a tumor is likely to be.

STAGING

Staging is a system of classifying all types of cancer according to features of the tumor, such as size and whether it has spread to the lymph nodes or to distant organs. *Clinical staging* includes physical examination, with careful inspection and palpation of the breast and the area surrounding it, including the lymph nodes. *Pathologic staging* includes: all the elements of clinical staging plus microscopic examination of the excised cancer and the margin of tissue around it; measurement of the size of the primary tumor; determination of whether the cancer has invaded the chest wall (including the ribs and the muscles between them); and evaluation of whether there is regional (armpit lymph nodes) or distant metastasis. Usually, the surgeon removes the axillary or underarm lymph nodes to complete this staging process. (Lymph nodes or glands are the small bean-shaped filters that join the lymphatic vessels. They also contain certain disease-fighting immune system cells.)

When staging was first developed more than sixty years ago, the one-step procedure was in common use. Because the woman was already undergoing an operation, it wasn't difficult for the surgeon to assess the lymph nodes at the same time the cancer was removed. Today, however, the two-step procedure is preferred, and staging may not be complete until the definitive second step is done.

If several lymph nodes contain cancer cells, there is a possibility that the cancer has spread to distant parts of the body, and the doctor typically recommends further diagnostic imaging tests. These may include a radionuclide scan of the bones and/or liver, computed tomography (CT or CAT scan), and/or magnetic resonance imaging (MRI).

Armed with the knowledge of the size of your primary tumor (T), the status of your lymph nodes (N), and whether there is metastasis (M), your doctor assigns a descriptive stage to your breast cancer, based on the TNM system established by the American Joint Committee on Cancer (AJCC).

Primary Tumor

Your physician can classify the size of your primary tumor as T1, T2, T3, or T4. Classifications of T0 to T1 require mammographic and/or pathologic examination. The following are descriptions of T0 through T4 stages, including subsets of T1 and T4:

TX   The primary tumor cannot be assessed.
T0   There is no evidence of a primary tumor.

Tis   Carcinoma in situ: intraductal carcinoma (DCIS), lobular
      carcinoma in situ (LCIS), or *Paget's disease*, which is a can-
      cer that involves the nipple and may not produce a tumor. If
      it does cause a tumor, the cancer is staged according to the
      size of the tumor.

T1   The tumor is 2 cm (centimeters; about 3/4 inch) or less at
      its greatest dimension.

    T1a   0.5 cm (slightly less than 1/4 inch) or less in its great-
      est dimension.

    T1b   More than 0.5 cm but not more than 1 cm in its great-
      est dimension.

    T1c   More than 1 cm but not more than 2 cm in its greatest
      dimension.

T2   The tumor is more than 2 cm but not more than 5 cm (2
      inches) at its greatest dimension.

T3   The tumor is more than 5 cm at its greatest dimension.

T4   A tumor of any size with extension to the chest wall or skin.

    T4a   Extension to chest wall.

    T4b   Edema (swelling) or ulceration (an open sore) of the
      breast skin or related skin nodules in the same breast.

    T4c   Both T4a and T4b.

    T4d   *Inflammatory carcinoma*, a kind of breast cancer that
      involves the skin, sometimes causing it to turn red and
      thicken. A lump usually cannot be felt in the breast
      tissue.

Regional Lymph Nodes

Almost all of the lymphatic vessels of the breast drain to the *axillary lymph nodes* under the arm, along the axillary vein on the
same side of the body. There is very little drainage to the *internal
mammary nodes*, which are along the space where the ribs join

the breastbone. When cancer spreads beyond these two areas of lymph nodes, it is considered distant metastatic cancer (M1). The following are stages that apply to *ipsilateral* lymph nodes — those on the same side of the body as the breast with cancer:

NX Regional lymph nodes cannot be assessed.

N0 No regional lymph node spread.

N1 Ipsilateral axillary lymph node(s) are involved, but the nodes are movable.

N2 Ipsilateral axillary lymph node(s) are involved and are fixed to one another or to other structures.

N3 Ipsilateral internal mammary lymph node(s) are involved.

Lymph nodes can also be described according to the number and size of the nodes involved.

Distant Metastasis

Breast cancer can spread to nearly every part of the body, but the most common sites, in order of frequency, are: bone, lung, liver, and brain. Stage of metastasis, including spread to lymph nodes beyond the breast region, is indicated as follows:

MX Presence of distant metastasis cannot be assessed.

M0 No distant metastasis.

M1 Distant metastasis.

Stage Groupings

By combining the three categories described above, physicians indicate one general stage grouping. There are seven major stage groupings:

Stage 0	Tis	N0	M0
Stage I	T1	N0	M0
StageIIA	T0	N1	M0
	T1	N1	M0
	T2	N0	M0
Stage IIB	T2	N1	M0
	T3	N0	M0
Stage IIIA	T0	N2	M0
	T1	N2	M0
	T2	N2	M0
	T3	N1	M0
	T3	N2	M0
Stage IIIB	T4	Any N	M0
	Any T	N3	M0
Stage IV	Any T	Any N	M1

For example a 2.5 cm tumor with no lymph node involvement and no metastasis present is a Stage IIA breast cancer. When breast cancer has spread to a distant site, such as the lung, it is Stage IV.

Knowing the stage of your cancer is important when you begin to evaluate treatment recommendations and survival rates. The suggested treatment options for each stage are available through the National Cancer Institute's Physicians Data Query (PDQ) (see the Resources section following Chapter 2). Your doctor's suggested approach for your stage of cancer may mirror that given the PDQ or differ from it. If it varies from the current standard, you should understand why. And if you do any research on your own, you will see that the stage of disease is an important predictor of survival. It's also a major factor that researchers use in designing studies and comparing treatment results.

TREATMENT OPTIONS

Never feel rushed to make a decision. You have about three weeks to gather information, talk to breast surgeons and medical and radiation oncologists, and research your treatment options. It's always better to get a second opinion from a doctor who has no relationship to the first doctor you've seen. The doctor you're consulting for a second opinion will then analyze your case from the beginning, not taking into consideration the first doctor's recommendation. After consulting with one or more doctors, you'll need to decide who should treat you, what treatment you will have, and where you will have it. Sometimes, the decision is easy. You talk to two doctors, they both agree, they're at medical institutions with good reputations, and your choice becomes primarily a matter of convenience and personality. But the decisions can be far more complicated.

Perhaps you have several treatment options. One is complicated, perhaps even risky; another is established but inconvenient. One conserves the breast; another doesn't. And then there's the issue of costs. What does your health care plan permit? What will your insurance cover? Some choices are appealing but difficult to find or arrange in your area. Are you willing to travel? How important is it to have your family nearby? The best way to avoid being overwhelmed by the choices, not to mention the research involved in coming to a decision, is to break the task down into manageable parts, beginning with gathering your personal information.

Keeping Track of Your Records

If you see only one surgeon and follow his or her advice for treatment, you know that all your records are in your file, and your biopsy is stored in one laboratory. However, if you want a second opinion or think you may want to consult with another doctor in the future, you need to keep copies of all your laboratory reports and X-rays.

You will need a duplicate of your mammogram and a copy of the radiologist's report. Request a copy of any reports on other tests, including blood tests and scans that are part of your diagnostic workup, from the doctor who orders them. Ask for the tissue slides of your tumor and a copy of the pathologist's report. Laboratories differ in their policies regarding slides. Some will give slides directly to you, but all will agree to send them to a physician of your choice. Laboratories always keep blocks of your tissue so that recuts or duplicates can be made if necessary.

Write a clear, concise outline of your own medical history. Provide important details such as previous operations, childbirths, major ailments, chronic diseases, drugs taken for prolonged periods as well as any medication you are currently taking (including vitamins, oral contraceptives, and estrogen replacement therapy) or to which you are allergic, and anything in your family history that may be significant, such as whether your parents or siblings have cancer. If possible, print or type this so that it can be easily read.

HOW SHOULD THE TUMOR BE REMOVED?

The breast specialist who did your biopsy will have a recommendation for the definitive surgery—possibly removing the tumor and assessing whether your lymph nodes are involved (see Chapter 7). If the surgeon believes you have Stage 0 (intraductal) breast cancer, a lumpectomy or, in a case of widespread disease, a total mastectomy are two possibilities. If you have Stage I or II cancer, the recommendation almost always involves a lumpectomy and axillary lymph node removal or a modified radical mastectomy. Additional treatments such as radiation and chemotherapy will also be discussed. The doctor can be fairly certain of all the possibilities, but no final recommendation can be made until after surgery, when the lymph nodes can be assessed and the stage of disease can be determined.

Whenever you seek a second opinion, be fully prepared, and take your X-rays (mammograms), slides, and reports with you. The second doctor may agree with your first doctor's recommendation or make other suggestions. If the two physicians express different opinions, you may want to seek a third or even a fourth opinion. In most cases, after two or three consultations, you will have a good idea of your options and the advantages and disadvantages of each.

It's also important to weigh the pros and cons of where you will be treated. If you don't live close to a big city, you may prefer to be treated by a nearby surgeon in a community hospital. Today, many community hospitals can offer high-quality care. However, being treated in a teaching institution offers several advantages— for example, access to several different specialists, from radiologists to social workers, under one roof. If your cancer is advanced or is complicated in any way, it's almost always better to be treated in a hospital that provides *multidisciplinary* care—specialists in diagnosis, surgery, radiation therapy, and chemotherapy are available. Many university-associated institutions now have centers devoted solely to the diagnosis and treatment of breast cancer. Along with knowledgeable care, these centers often offer convenience. You can schedule visits with more than one doctor on the same morning or afternoon, and take advantage of the center's nonmedical support services that are specifically directed to your needs and can be of great value.

Your choices may, of course, be limited by your HMO's health care plan. Opinions on treatments outside of your plan, for example, may be at your own cost.

THE FINAL DECISION

The components of the therapy that your doctors present to you are designed to achieve local control, regional control, and body-wide or systemic control of the disease. *Local control* means using surgery or radiation therapy, or both, to remove or destroy cancer cells in the breast tissue and prevent a recurrence of cancer. *Regional control* includes treatment directed to the axillary lymph nodes. (Regional control is sometimes considered with local control.) *Systemic control*, which is accomplished through chemotherapy and/or hormone therapy, means preventing the spread of the disease and destroying cancer cells that may have migrated to distant parts of the body.

If your breast cancer is advanced at the time of surgery, you are forced to make more complex decisions than someone who has a small localized cancer with no lymph nodes involved. But all women with breast cancer at any stage have the same general principle to consider: What treatments will give local/regional and systemic control? These can be thought of as almost two separate issues.

The following questions may help you when you talk about your treatment options with your doctor. (You may find it useful to first read Chapters 7 through 9, on surgery, radiation therapy, and chemotherapy, respectively.)

1. What are the chances of long-term survival with the suggested therapy? In most cases, the survival rates of the

different types of surgery are similar. For example, for women with Stage I and Stage II breast cancer who are candidates for breast-conserving treatment, the long-term survival rates—about 80 percent—are the same as for breast-conserving treatment and mastectomy.

2. What are the chances that the cancer will come back, and what are your options if that happens?

3. Which follow-up treatments and procedures are necessary? For example, lumpectomy usually requires six weeks of five-days-a-week radiation therapy; mastectomy for Stages 0 to II usually does not. For some women, the daily trips to the radiology facility are simply too inconvenient or too tiring.

4. What are the psychological issues involved in each option? Is fear of recurrence a serious issue for you? What does the loss of a breast mean to your self-esteem? Your sexuality? Will the surgery affect your ability to function in any way?

Research has shown that, in terms of overall emotional distress, women who have a mastectomy do not suffer more emotionally than women who have breast-conserving surgery. However, women who have breast-conserving treatment (see Chapter 8) and no mastectomy seem to have a more positive attitude about their body image, and their sense of their sexual desirability remains unchanged.

Chapter 7

Surgery

Without any doubt, surgical removal of cancer from the breast is the most important and sometimes the only treatment for breast cancer. The extent of the surgery—usually ranging from lumpectomy (removal of the tumor alone) to modified radical mastectomy (removal of the breast and underarm lymph nodes)—depends on several factors: the size of the cancer relative to the size of the breast; whether the cancer has spread to the lymph nodes—and which ones; and whether the cancer has spread to the muscles beneath the breast. Radical mastectomy (removal of the breast, underarm lymph nodes, and chest muscle) is very rarely done nowadays.

By the time surgery is scheduled, the surgeons who examined your breast and reviewed your tests, including your biopsy report, have a good idea of the size and aggressiveness of your cancer. Their recommendation for surgery is based on these factors and on their estimate of the stage of your cancer. Opinions vary; if the doctors you consulted have different recommendations, you will have to decide whose advice you will follow.

When you consult with surgeons, keep in mind that there are several objectives. The main concern is to remove enough tissue to control the cancer and lower the risk of a recurrence, and to do so in an operation that causes you minimal disfigurement and disability. Surgeons nearly always remove some lymph nodes

from under the arm nearest the breast, and order a biopsy procedure called *axillary dissection*. The extent of this surgery is controversial and depends on the extent of the cancer in the breast,
but the procedure is usually done so that the lymph nodes can be
checked under a microscope to see if they contain any cancer
cells. Knowing whether lymph nodes are involved is necessary for
identifying the stage of the disease and for avoiding cancer growth
in the underarm area. Lymph node dissection is almost never performed in intraductal (Stage 0) breast cancer.

Before you have an operation of any kind, your surgeon will
describe the planned surgery in detail, mention other procedures
that may be necessary if something unexpected is discovered, and
discuss the possible risks and complications of the surgery and the
anesthesia—all as part of the informed consent process. As with
certain diagnostic tests, you will be asked to sign a document indicating that you have been informed about the surgery and are
consenting to it.

TYPES OF SURGERY

Breast-conserving surgery is the removal of a tumor and a margin
of tissue around it. You will sometimes hear the term *breast-
conserving treatment* (see page 89), which indicates breast-
conserving surgery, usually with removal of some lymph nodes,
followed by a course of radiation therapy. Depending on the size
of the tumor, breast-conserving surgery may consist of only a
lumpectomy or, if more breast tissue is removed, a *partial* or *segmental mastectomy*. A *quadrantectomy* is the removal of one-
fourth of the breast, but it is categorized as breast-conserving
surgery. Because doctors and nurses sometimes use these terms
interchangeably, ask your doctors exactly what they mean by the

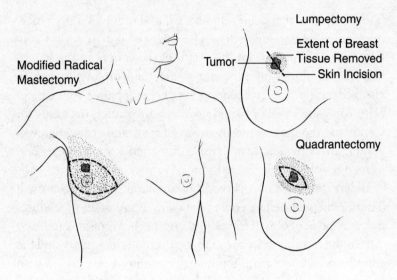

Figure 7.1: Surgical treatments for breast cancer.

term they use to describe your case and how much breast tissue they are expecting to remove. (See Figure 7.1.)

When none of the breast tissue can be preserved, the operation falls under the broad category of *mastectomy*. A *simple* or *total mastectomy* is defined as removal of all the breast, including the nipple and areola, but not the lymph nodes.

In a *subcutaneous mastectomy*, the breast tissue is excised from beneath the skin, but the nipple and areola are not removed. If enough breast tissue is removed from beneath the nipple, it becomes insensitive; if enough breast tissue is saved to preserve sensation, then the purpose of mastectomy is defeated. Therefore, this procedure is almost never performed for cancer.

A *modified radical mastectomy*, which is a total mastectomy plus removal of the axillary lymph nodes, is very common. This procedure can be pictured as a breast amputation: the breast is removed, but much of the overlying skin and all of the underlying muscle are preserved. It is possible to reconstruct the missing breast mound immediately after a mastectomy, or months or even years later (see "Reconstruction," pages 88–110).

A *radical mastectomy* removes not only the breast but also the pectoralis major or chest muscle beneath the breast and all the lymph nodes under the arm. It is rarely done today unless a very large tumor is present or the cancer involves the chest wall. However, if your mother or grandmother had this type of operation many years go, you probably noticed that the chest area where her breast would have been was sunken with great deformity. Women who have this extensive surgery have difficulty being fitted for a prosthesis. If this procedure is necessary today, reconstruction is possible but usually requires several operations and the cosmetic result is limited.

BREAST-CONSERVING TREATMENT (BCT)

For early-stage cancer (Stage I or II), breast-conserving treatment (BCT) has become the current standard of care. Several large studies compared women who had BCT with women who had mastectomies and found that the ten-year survival rates are the same. Researchers have also studied women who underwent one of these operations in the more distant past and found that those who had BCT had low rates of cancer recurrence. The women were also satisfied with the cosmetic results of the surgery.

In June 1990, a Consensus Development Conference on the Treatment of Early-Stage Breast Cancer, convened by the National Cancer Institute, came to the following conclusion:

Breast conservation treatment is an appropriate method of primary therapy for the majority of women with Stage I and II breast cancer and is preferable because it provides survival equivalent to total mastectomy and axillary dissection while preserving the breast.

Today, a woman with early-stage breast cancer is offered a choice of a modified radical mastectomy or a lumpectomy plus radiation therapy.

There is little debate about whether radiation therapy is needed after lumpectomy, but several studies are being done in an attempt to define the minority who do not need radiation therapy and are not likely to develop cancer again. At this time, those studies are not conclusive.

Is BCT for You?

If the cancer is small relative to the size of your breasts, you are a candidate for breast-conserving treatment. You must have a diagnostic mammogram before the final decision is made. Along with assessing the size and extent of your tumor, the purpose of the mammogram is to discover any other abnormalities that cannot be felt in the breast with cancer or in the opposite one. The surgeon also examines the skin for any thickening over the tumor, which might indicate extension of the cancer. The mammogram may be magnified, for precise examination. A "cone" view is a view focused on one area to locate an abnormality. If it is not possible to feel the abnormality, a dye may be injected, or, more commonly, a very thin wire is placed in the breast and an X-ray is taken to ensure that the tiny area is accurately pinpointed for surgery.

The Procedure

You may receive a general anesthetic to make you unconscious during the surgery. More typically, you will be given an intravenous sedative to make you drowsy and a local anesthetic to deaden the nerves in the breast. The surgeon will usually make a curved incision just above the tumor; a slight scar will form eventually. Two curved incisions that meet at either end to form an oval may be necessary, and a slightly more obvious scar may result when the ellipse of skin is removed. Rarely is it necessary to remove large areas of skin.

The surgeon removes the tumor and a margin of surrounding tissue. Tiny metal clips are placed in the breast tissue to mark the area that will be receiving extra radiation therapy. The wound is closed with sutures. Depending on the location of the tumor and the amount of tissue removed, the surgeon may bring the edges of the tissue under the skin together with dissolvable sutures and then close the incision with dissolvable or removable stitches. The appearance of the breast after BCT will depend greatly on how much tissue is removed. Some women with small breasts find it necessary to wear a special bra, so that the breast that has had surgery matches the size of the opposite one.

After the lump is removed, the surgeon makes a separate incision in the underarm and removes several lymph nodes for study. (The size of the tumor and certain other characteristics determine the number of lymph nodes sampled.) If the tumor is in the area of breast tissue that extends to the underarm, or in the upper, outer quadrant of the breast, the cancer and some lymph nodes can be removed through the same incision.

After examining the tissue removed during the surgery, the pathologist will describe in a report where the tissue came from, the size of the tissue removed, and the size of the breast cancer. He or she will note the histologic type and grade of the tumor, will do an analysis of the hormone receptors and will note whether or not the cancer has spread to the blood vessels or lymph vessels. Finally, tissue from the margins surrounding the tumor will be examined to search for cancer cells. If more are discovered, the surgeon will often operate again, soon after the first operation, to remove another margin of tissue. This is called a *re-excision lumpectomy*. The pathologist also notes how many lymph nodes are affected, if any.

Who Cannot Have BCT?

Breast-conserving treatment may be ruled out entirely, or discouraged, if you have any of the following conditions:

1. You are pregnant. The surgery isn't a problem, but the radiation therapy that follows would endanger the developing baby. If you are in the late months of your pregnancy when the cancer is discovered, it may be possible to postpone the radiation therapy until after you deliver. However, this would be considered experimental; most pregnant women are treated with mastectomy.
2. You have cancer in more than one area of the breast, or there are suspicious lesions or microcalcifications throughout the breast.
3. You have received radiation therapy to the breast in the past. The breast tissue cannot withstand another course of radiation without becoming seriously damaged.
4. You have a history of collagen vascular disease. People with diseases such as lupus erythematosus and scleroderma may not be able to tolerate the radiation therapy.
5. Your breast is small and the tumor is large. In this case, the cosmetic alteration is too great.
6. You have very large breasts. BCT is a possibility for you, but the radiation therapy may require special equipment.
7. You are not willing to undergo radiation therapy.

8. The tumor is directly under the nipple, or removal of the tumor alone removes part of the nipple and areola. In either case, the cosmetic result can make BCT less appealing.

LYMPH NODE DISSECTION

Axillary lymph node dissection or *lymphadenectomy* is removal of the lymph nodes under the arm. The main goal in removing the lymph nodes for microscopic examination is determining the stage of the cancer and deciding whether systemic treatment, such as chemotherapy or hormonal therapy, is necessary. If the lymph nodes do contain cancer cells, removing them is also a form of regional treatment aimed at controlling cancer in the axilla. If staging will not make a difference in terms of systemic treatment, and the lymph nodes appear normal, then the necessity of removing the lymph nodes must be reconsidered.

Over the years, there has been a continuing debate about the benefit of routinely removing the axillary lymph nodes in women who have small cancers but no evidence of cancer spread. In about half the women who have lymph node dissection, there is no cancer spread, which leads some experts who oppose routine lymph node dissection to say the procedure puts some women at unnecessary risk for chronic swelling of the arm, nerve damage, or other complications of the surgery. The methods currently used to determine who needs the surgery and who doesn't are being studied. Meanwhile, the only infallible method for learning whether the lymph nodes are involved is to remove them.

Efforts to resolve the issue have had shortcomings that make the results questionable. Some years ago, two British studies showed that breast cancer was less likely to recur, and survival increased, among those who received axillary dissection. However, because the women in the study had different types of surgery, it is possible that the benefits were not related to the lymph node removal. A larger, more recent study in France showed a similar benefit, but it cannot be known whether the higher rate of survival was due to the lymph node removal or to chemotherapy, which was given to the women who had cancer in lymph nodes discovered when these nodes were removed. In Denmark, a study of more than 3,000 women showed that breast cancer recurrence was higher and five-year survival rates were lower in women who had fewer than five lymph nodes removed. In the United States, the National Surgical Adjuvant Breast Protocol (NSABP) trial attempted to resolve the debate. The subjects of the study were about 1,000 women with breast cancer who did not appear to have lymph node involvement preoperatively, when examined physically. One group received mastectomies that included removal of the axillary lymph nodes; another group was supposed to have had total mastectomies with no lymph node removal. After ten years, there was no significant difference in survival, but, unfortunately, the study was flawed: 35 percent of the women who received total mastectomy as the only treatment did have some lymph nodes removed. (This can happen because the top of the breast and the lower portion of the lymph nodes intersect.) And, even though all the women appeared to have no cancer in their lymph nodes at the outset, almost 20 percent of them without axillary dissection had the cancer grow back in the underarm lymph nodes. Furthermore, not enough women were enrolled for a statistically significant benefit to be detected.

Experts continue to debate the pros and cons of lymph node dissection, but a strong case can be made for the surgery. Given the large number of women who are diagnosed with breast cancer each year, if lymph node dissection improves the survival time in only 5 to 10 percent of them, the procedure is still helping a great many women.

The whole question would be moot if there was an accurate way to assess lymph node involvement without surgery and remove the nodes from only those women whose cancer had spread. A new technique called *lymph node mapping and sentinel lymph node biopsy* may resolve the problem. Researchers studying the function of lymph nodes discovered that one node may be affected by cancer before the others. If this *sentinel node* contains cancer cells, then other nodes may also be involved; if the sentinel node is free of cancer, the others are almost certainly free of cancer also.

Sentinel lymph node mapping has been used successfully for several years for melanoma, a serious skin cancer. The technique is somewhat more difficult to apply to an internal organ such as the breast. In this procedure, a radioactive tracer and/or a blue dye is injected near the tumor. The dye or radioactive material is carried by the lymphatic vessels to a sentinel node, which is detected by the surgeon in the operating room who can see the blue dye and/or localize the radioactive material with a geiger counter. Studies are in progress to determine in which patients a sentinel lymph node biopsy should be used routinely instead of an axillary dissection. If your surgeon is considering this procedure, it might be useful to ask how many sentinel node biopsies he/she has done, and whether this approach will be part of a research study. If this technique is not performed expertly the patient may be harmed by undertreatment of her breast cancer. For example, it is possible to retrieve a noncancerous lymph node and inaccurately call it the sentinal node, while the true sentinal node and perhaps other lymph nodes, actually contain cancer that will be undetected. In this situation, the patient would receive no surgery to remove the cancerous lymph nodes and would have less than optimal chemotherapy, probably reducing her chance for a cure.

MASTECTOMY

Your physician will recommend a mastectomy if you have a large tumor, if there is more than one malignant tumor in your breast, or if you have clusters of suspicious microcalcifications throughout your breast, particularly when a biopsy of one or more indicates a malignancy. If none of these conditions exists, your doctor may still suggest mastectomy for other reasons. For instance, perhaps mastectomy is the treatment that the doctor is most experienced with and has the most confidence in. If you have early-stage breast cancer, ask your surgeon why he or she is suggesting mastectomy instead of BCT.

To some degree, knowing that a mastectomy is the only option eliminates the stress of making a treatment decision, but you still face the physical stress and emotional upheaval of having a major, body-altering operation. Women who have had mastectomies say they found it helpful to share their concerns and feelings with those close to them, and studies have shown that women who have a supportive circle of family or friends, or who participate in a support group of strangers, recover more quickly, both physically and emotionally.

The extent of a mastectomy depends on the size of the tumor, whether it is attached to the chest wall, and whether it has spread to any nearby lymph nodes. Some of these conditions cannot be known until the operation is under way, but you can discuss their likelihood with your surgeon beforehand. Remember: the object is to remove all the cancer while keeping disfigurement and disability to a minimum.

The Procedure

You will be under general anesthesia for the operation, which can take from one to three hours. The technique discussed here generally applies to mastectomies that do not involve the chest muscle. A description of the extensive radical mastectomy, in which the chest muscle is removed, is given later in the chapter. A radical mastectomy is necessary in less than 5 percent of cases.

The surgeon performing a mastectomy typically makes two incisions that form an ellipse across the width of the breast. The skin within the oval, which includes the nipple and the previous biopsy incision, is removed, and the remaining skin over the breast is lifted so the surgeon can remove the underlying breast tissue. A thin layer of tissue covering the muscle of the chest wall beneath the breast is also removed. A surgeon performing a modified radical mastectomy will remove a cluster of lymph nodes under the arm. Lymph node removal or dissection is technically difficult; care must be taken to avoid injuring the major veins and nerves along the chest muscle and in the axilla.

The wound is stitched closed using sutures that will dissolve gradually. The surgeon places two tiny tubes, or drains, in the incision and under the skin. One of them will remove fluid from the underarm area. (These will be removed when drainage through the tube stops, usually about the same time the stitches are removed.) Then the chest is bandaged with a tight dressing or surgical bra, and a small gauze dressing is placed over the underarm incision.

While you are in the recovery room, a nurse monitors your vital signs and checks the bandage and drains frequently to be sure there is no excessive bleeding.

Your surgeon will check on you in the recovery room. When you are fully conscious and aware of your surroundings, he or she may talk to you about the operation and report on the pathologist's early findings, if any have become available. When the pathologist has completed the microscopic studies—which may take as long as five to seven days—and you are in better shape to

EARLY DISCHARGE

The length of a hospital stay after a mastectomy is usually two days, unless reconstructive surgery takes place immediately afterward. The time you need to be hospitalized is based on your condition, the type of surgery you have, whether there is someone who can care for you at home, how comfortable you are, and whether there are any other health problems or complications following the surgery. Regardless of the many possible adverse situations, some managed-care plans have encouraged doctors to discharge mastectomy patients on the day of surgery.

This *ambulatory mastectomy*—or "drive-by mastectomy," as some critics have called it—is very controversial. Physicians and their patients cite pain after surgery, fear of postoperative bleeding and infection, and difficulty dealing with the drains and dressings as just a few of the concerns that make early discharge problematic.

Health insurers acknowledge that ambulatory mastectomy is not for every woman, but they maintain that, with good education beforehand, some women are actually more comfortable being cared for at home. Nevertheless, for the health insurers, early discharge is a money-saving issue. At this time, no studies have been done to determine how often same-day discharged women have had to return to a hospital because of hemorrhage or pain, but it is unlikely that ambulatory mastectomy will become the rule.

discuss your condition and ask questions, you can go over the details of the pathologist's report with your doctor(s).

In very rare circumstances, when cancer is detected at an advanced stage and involves the chest wall, the surgeon may recommend a radical mastectomy to remove all the breast tissue and lymph nodes plus the muscles that separate the breast from the rib cage. This extensive surgery requires a longer recovery time than a total mastectomy and should be followed by physical therapy to regain function of the arm and shoulder. (See Figure 7.2.)

COMPLICATIONS AND SIDE EFFECTS AFTER BREAST CANCER SURGERY

Complications and side effects are more common after radical surgery than after other types of mastectomies because the disruption to the tissues is so much greater. The discomfort and complications following a mastectomy or a lumpectomy are largely due to the removal of lymph nodes under the arm. The greater the number of lymph nodes removed, the more uncomfortable the recovery period is likely to be, and the greater the chance of complications. In a radical mastectomy, *all* the lymph nodes near the diseased breast are removed.

FLUID BUILDUP

Immediately after surgery, blood and tissue fluid begin collecting under the mastectomy skin flaps, and lymph begins collecting at the lymph node site. The surgeon therefore places a tiny temporary drain into the wound and makes a stitch or two to hold it in place. The fluid flowing through this drain collects in a small, lightweight, closed plastic reservoir. As much as three or four ounces of fluid can seep through the temporary drain each day. The amount will gradually diminish over the next several days. As healing begins, the color of the fluid changes from red-tinged to clear yellow. (It should not be bright red. If it is, call your doctor immediately. This is a sign that there is some internal bleeding and the wound is not healing properly.) Before you leave the hospital, you should be taught how to empty the drain collection device and what signs of trouble to watch for. The drain is typically removed when no more than an ounce of fluid accumulates in twenty-four hours.

Despite the preventive step of having a drain in place, about 15 percent of women develop a *seroma*—an accumulation of too much fluid in a small area that feels something like a squishy lump or a foam-rubber ball. Not only is this uncomfortable, but it can interfere with healing and lead to infection. See a doctor or nurse, who can withdraw the fluid through a syringe. The procedure isn't painful, but it may need to be repeated. In rare instances another drain may be inserted in an attempt to facilitate the flow of fluid.

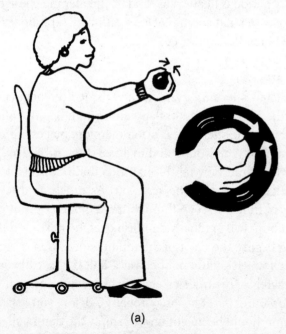

(a)

Figure 7.2: Exercises recommended after mastectomy.

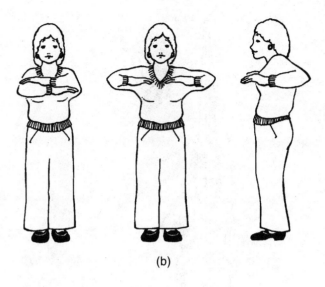

(b)

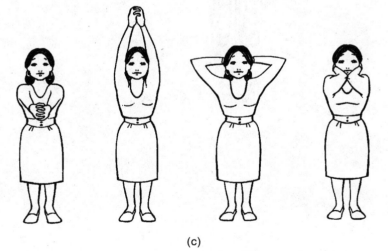

(c)

Figure 7.2: Continued.

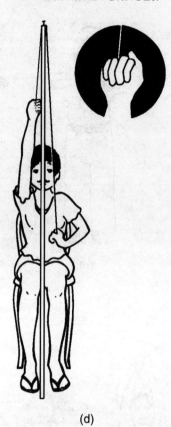

(d)

Figure 7.2: Continued.

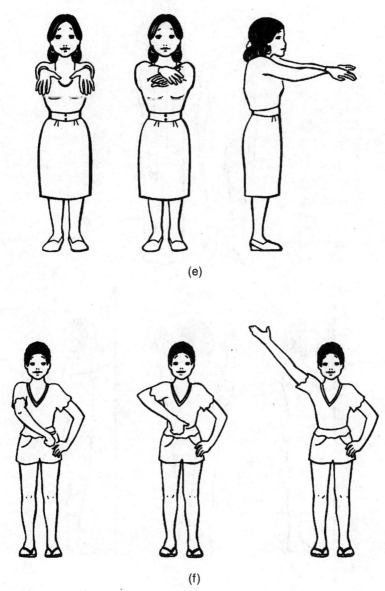

(e)

(f)

Figure 7.2: Continued.

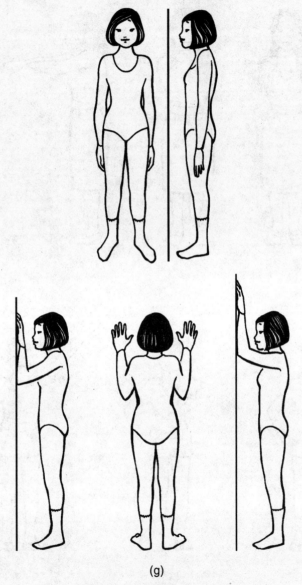

(g)

Figure 7.2: Continued.

The drain may accomplish the job of removing fluid from the underarm, but it can still be uncomfortable. Some women describe being conscious of the drain as something unusual under the skin.

SWELLING

After surgery to remove lymph nodes, the flow of lymph fluid can be partially interrupted. Eventually, lymph vessels adjacent to the area will drain lymph fluid away, but the transition doesn't always go smoothly. Scarring, lymph vessel damage from radiation therapy, and infection can add to the blockage, and some degree of swelling may occur.

Swelling of the arm, or *lymphedema*, ranges from mild, in which the arm close to the surgery site is 1 to 1.5 centimeters (about a half-inch) larger in circumference than the other, to severe, in which the arm is more than 5 centimeters larger. Lymphedema, the most common postoperative complication, occurs some time after axillary lymph node surgery. It may take a month or two to develop; in some women, it occurs many years later. As many as 10 percent of women who have mastectomies eventually have lymphedema. There are some preventive activities, such as raising the surgery-side arm periodically throughout the day, and sleeping with that arm elevated on a pillow at night. If the arm has a tendency to swell, a special compression sleeve can be worn to provide necessary support and prevent fluid from accumulating. Other precautions that are helpful are: avoiding infection; mild, range-of-motion exercises; massage; avoiding carrying heavy objects; avoiding strain; and wearing loose sleeves.

Because the lymphatic vessels have been cut and the nodes removed, there is a lifelong risk of lymphedema. If you haven't been taught ways to prevent swelling, ask your doctor or nurse to

PREVENTING LYMPHEDEMA

To prevent lymphedema, the American Cancer Society recommends protecting the arm from injury in the following ways:

1. Protect your fingers from punctures by sharp objects, such as needles and pins.
2. Care for simple cuts, scratches, or burns by carefully washing them and covering them with a protective dressing. Be sure to change plastic wound wraps or bandages often, to avoid infection.
3. Wear loose-fitting gloves and avoid wearing anything that will constrict your hand or arm, such as tight sleeves or jewelry.
4. Inform laboratory technicians, nurses, and doctors of your surgery and of the need for care in taking blood pressure or having vaccinations or injections on the affected arm or hand.
5. Manicure your fingernails carefully. Avoid cutting or tearing cuticles; use cream to keep them soft.
6. When gardening, protect your hand and arm by wearing gloves thick enough to protect against punctures from thorns or injuries from tools.
7. Protect your arm and chest from the sun, particularly if you have received radiation therapy. When you will be in bright sunlight, wear protective clothing and apply an SPF-15 (or higher) sunscreen liberally to exposed areas.

explain them to you on your first postoperative visit. The main preventive strategy is to avoid infection.

PAIN AND SENSITIVITY

The pain experienced after breast surgery varies, depending on the extent of the operation. Within a week after surgery, a mild pain medicine at bedtime is usually all that is needed. Increasing discomfort, however, can be a warning that healing is not progressing as it should or that a seroma or infection is present. Let your doctor know.

Another kind of sensitivity comes from having the nerves under the arm cut or damaged when the lymph nodes are removed. Some women complain of numbness or heaviness in the arm on the side where the nodes were removed. Others feel a burning sensation or a tingling like "pins and needles." Some women don't notice any change in sensation. Women who have a lumpectomy may experience a numbness under the incision. And some women who have had a mastectomy say that they feel discomfort or sensations like itching in the breast that was removed, even though it's no longer there. Called *phantom* sensation, this pain is caused by the former nerve connections, and it will eventually diminish. Some women also complain of a "tight" feeling in their chest. All of these unpleasant sensations do fade, but they may take as long as a year to disappear entirely.

INFECTION

About 10 to 15 percent of women who have mastectomies or lymph node removal develop some type of early complication. Infection is the most troublesome problem, and seroma (see above) is the most common. An increase in redness or tenderness along the incision; swelling of the arm, the chest, or armpit; or pus around where the drain enters the wound or along the incision—any of these conditions indicates a possible infection. So does a temperature above 101 degrees Fahrenheit. Report any of these symptoms to your doctor at once.

There will always be some risk of infection in your arm if you had lymph nodes removed. Make the precautions listed in "Preventing Lymphedema," on page 106, your daily habits.

RECONSTRUCTION

Breast reconstruction surgery has become so refined that it can be accomplished in almost every woman who has a mastectomy. Today, about one-third of those who have a breast removed choose to have it rebuilt using their own tissue (*autologous tissue*) or reconstructed with an implant. Most implants are circular silicone envelopes filled with saline or silicone gel or both.

Even women who have a lumpectomy may benefit from reconstruction if so much breast tissue has been excised that the treated breast is noticeably smaller than the healthy one. However, there are several shortcomings of reconstruction after lumpectomy. For example, lumpectomy is usually followed with a course of radiation therapy, and tissue that has been irradiated has more difficulty healing. Also, an implant behind the breast may not restore the post-lumpectomy breast contour very well, because the tissue is missing in only one area. At this time, there is no such thing as an implant that can be made to match the size and shape of tissue removed in a lumpectomy, and an implant cannot be placed into the breast but only under it.

Reconstructive surgery can be done immediately after the cancer surgery (*immediate reconstruction*) or at some time after healing from the mastectomy is complete (*delayed reconstruction*). Some women and their doctors prefer immediate reconstruction because it may lessen the emotional impact of the mastectomy. However, when mastectomy and reconstruction are done at the same time, the operation is longer and there is an increased chance of wound-healing problems. You and your doctors will have to weigh the risks against the benefits for you. In general, if chemotherapy is part of the treatment plan, surgeons are more likely to recommend delayed reconstruction. They also take into account the size and location of the cancer, which determine the amount of skin to be removed in the mastectomy, but they are particularly concerned with other health factors such as age, obesity, and whether the woman smokes or has diabetes.

The goal of reconstructive surgery is to create a breast that matches the healthy breast. Occasionally, that requires reducing the size of the opposite, healthy breast—especially in women with very large breasts—or inserting an implant to enhance a smaller breast. Some women may find that a breast lift of the healthy breast gives a more balanced, symmetrical contour.

Women who are pleased with the results of breast reconstruction (most who have it are at least satisfied) say the procedure helped counter some of the mastectomy's negative effects on their sense of well-being and their self-image regarding their femininity and sexual desirability. In making the decision to have the operation, they considered practical aspects, such as not wanting to wear an external prosthesis and having more freedom in choosing clothing, as well as emotional concerns, such as wanting to feel less sexually inhibited. Whatever motivates the desire for breast reconstruction, studies show that most women are happy with the results, even when several operations are necessary to achieve a natural-appearing breast.

But reconstruction isn't for everyone. Women who choose not to have reconstruction feel just as comfortable with their decision as those who undergo the surgery. Women who reject reconstruction say they simply don't want additional surgery, especially when it sometimes involves multiple procedures. They believe that reconstruction presents too many risks or is too frightening, and that nothing really replaces a breast. Some fear there will be complications. And some say no because they feel comfortable wearing a breast prosthesis. Breast reconstruction can be thought of as merely an internal prosthesis. In general, older women are much less likely to have reconstruction because it involves more operative time and more complications because of their age.

As with any surgery, it's important to get at least one other opinion about the method and timing of your reconstructive surgery. It's also helpful to talk to women who have had the procedure planned for you. Ask about their experience with the benefits and drawbacks of reconstruction. The American Cancer Society's Reach to Recovery program, listed in the Resources section, can help you arrange a meeting with a woman who has had the surgery that you are contemplating.

Research indicates that most women know at the time of their cancer surgery whether they want reconstruction. This is good timing because it enables you to enlist a plastic surgeon as part of the treatment team and incorporate his or her opinion into surgical and recovery decisions. Something as basic as the location of the incision for an open biopsy can have an impact later if a mastectomy is to be followed by reconstructive surgery.

If you don't know whether you want to undergo this additional surgery, there's no harm in waiting. Some women undergo reconstructive surgery years after a mastectomy and are satisfied with the results. In fact, for some women, it's better to postpone the decision. Women who have a delayed reconstruction learn what living with a mastectomy is like, and they make their decision based on that knowledge. Those who have an immediate reconstruction never know whether they would have been more comfortable living with the appearance of a mastectomy than enduring the additional operations. In 1998, insurance coverage for breast reconstruction is very uncertain. Some companies cover the initial procedure, but not the operations that are needed to refine the results. Be sure to check with your insurer before making your final decision. And be aware that the costs can vary greatly; if there are complications, without insurance, the hospital bill can be as much as $15,000 to $20,000.

IMPLANTS

The oldest and simplest method of reconstructing the breast is to create a mound with a synthetic implant. The surgeon inserts the implant through the mastectomy incision and under the pectoralis major (chest) muscle. Occasionally, the surgeon may insert the implant through a new incision on the side of the breast nearest the armpit.

Implant Types

Many different sizes of implants and some slightly differently shaped ones are available today. Each type has advantages and disadvantages. On the sole basis of appearance, women with small-to-medium rounded breasts have the best chance of having their implant match their healthy breast.

There is some medical and legal controversy about the safety of silicone gel implants. Many women prefer them to saline-filled implants because the silicone feels more like breast tissue, and the gel shifts with movement more naturally. However, if a leak occurs, saline is absorbed into the body and is harmless. It has been questioned whether silicone can trigger certain connective tissue and autoimmune conditions (diseases in which the body's immune system attacks normal tissues). In 1992, the Food and Drug Administration (FDA) restricted the use of silicone implants in order to study the question. Women who desired reconstruction with silicone-filled implants after mastectomy were given access to clinical trials. Studies have not shown any increased risk of autoimmune disease among women with silicone implants. As a result, several organizations, including the American Cancer Society, have petitioned the FDA to ease the restrictions. Other countries did not take silicone implants off the market and the situation that occurred in the United States may be a reflection of our unique medical-legal climate, which does not necessarily benefit the patient.

Implant Surgery

The actual surgery to insert any type of implant is relatively simple. When done at the time of a mastectomy, the reconstruction adds only about an hour to the surgery. There are extra drains in place, and recovery time is longer because of the additional time under anesthesia, but the care afterward is the same as for a mastectomy alone. Delayed reconstruction requires about an hour

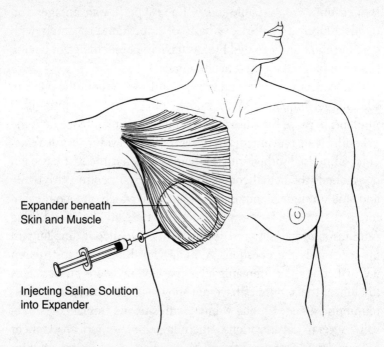

Expander beneath
Skin and Muscle

Injecting Saline Solution
into Expander

**Figure 7.3: Surgical implant of a tissue expander
after modified radical mastectomy.**

and a half. Drains are not routine, and recovery is much quicker than for immediate reconstruction because the mastectomy wound has already healed.

TISSUE EXPANDERS

The surgeon usually inserts a temporary tissue expander under the pectoralis muscle to stretch the muscle and the skin over the chest wall. The tissue expander is a silicone envelope with a valve-like opening or *port* through which a small amount of saline is injected. Every week or two, for one to three months, additional saline is injected until the expander is inflated to a size slightly larger than the implant will be. This gradual stretching feels similar to the stretching of the abdomen that occurs with pregnancy.

When the surrounding tissues are able to accommodate an implant and allow for a natural droop of the breast, the surgeon will replace the expander with a permanent implant. This is a thirty-minute operation that can be done on an outpatient basis. Usually, general anesthesia is used, but no overnight stay is required.

Some surgeons prefer an implant that combines the expander process with the permanent implant. After the skin expansion is complete, the filling valve is sealed. The expander remains in the breast as a permanent implant (Figure 7.3). The disadvantage of this type of implant is that the valve, which remains in place, may leak. Also, the permanent implant may need to be a slightly different shape.

COMPLICATIONS AND SIDE EFFECTS OF IMPLANTS

As with any surgery, there is a risk of postoperative infection, seroma (see page 100), and bleeding. Problems following reconstruction also include a loss of sensation in the breast; movement of the implant; breast *asymmetry*, or difference in the size and/or shape of the breasts; and *extrusion*, in which the implant begins to push out through the healing incision. The most common complication is a phenomenon known as *capsular contraction*, in which the pocket of scar tissue that forms around the implant becomes abnormally hard and can contract over the implant, causing the reconstructed breast to be misshapen.

Autologous Reconstruction

LATISSIMUS DORSI FLAP

If there is not enough skin to cover the implant, if the muscle over the chest wall has been removed, or if the skin has been so damaged by radiation that it cannot be stretched, the surgeon will remove a fan-shaped section of muscle and skin from the woman's

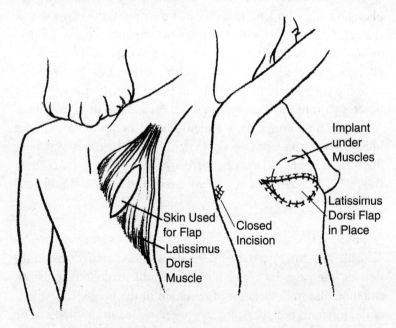

Figure 7.4: The latissimus dorsi flap procedure.

back, keeping the section attached to a portion of its own tissue, called a *pedicle*. The pedicle remains intact and contains the blood supply of the flap. This *latissimus dorsi flap*, which is named for the back muscle from which it comes, is tunneled under the skin, pulled out through an opening in the chest, and sutured in place over the mastectomy site (Figure 7.4). The surgeon then places an implant under the muscle to complete the reconstruction. The latissimus dorsi flap is virtually always a pedicle flap.

The latissimus dorsi flap procedure is obviously a much more complicated operation than an implant insertion. There is a scar on the woman's back, and there is a potential for shoulder problems because a portion of the muscle governing range of motion to the shoulder has been removed. There is about a 2 percent risk that a portion of the flap will not heal properly, and another operation may be necessary. However, this procedure usually creates a better result than when an implant is used alone, particularly in women with large breasts or women who have had radiation.

Several other surgical techniques use the body's own tissue to build a mound that feels and appears like a natural breast. The most common technique—the TRAM flap—carries its own blood supply. Another method—the free flap—requires meticulous and difficult microsurgery to connect tiny blood vessels in the flap to those in the chest wall.

TRAM FLAP

The TRAM flap uses tissue taken from the woman's abdomen (TRAM is an acronym for transverse rectus abdominis muscle). The surgery is complicated and time-consuming; it adds up to six hours to a mastectomy operation when the reconstruction is immediate.

A section of skin, underlying fat, and a portion of abdominal muscle are excised, leaving one or two pedicles of tissue with their natural blood supply. The flap is tunneled under the abdominal wall to the chest and rotated to fit the mastectomy wound. The edges of the breast incision are then sutured to the flap. (See Figure 7.5.)

Along with creating a breast with a natural texture, the technique gives the stomach a flatter appearance. However, some doctors caution against thinking of this as a "tummy tuck." Among the side effects not normally associated with that cosmetic procedure, some women experience abdominal weakness, sometimes to the point of being unable to do a situp. There is also an increased risk for developing an *abdominal hernia:* the abdominal organs may protrude through the weak area of muscle and form a bulge under the skin. The TRAM flap can be "sculpted" to match the shape of

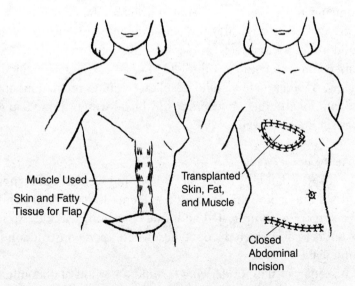

Muscle Used

Skin and Fatty
Tissue for Flap

Transplanted
Skin, Fat,
and Muscle

Closed
Abdominal
Incision

Figure 7.5: The TRAM flap procedure.

the other breast instead of leaving just the typical round shape of an implant.

The TRAM flap procedure is major surgery that may require a week in the hospital and another four to six weeks (or longer) of recovery at home. Women who smoke usually cannot have this operation; they are likely to develop healing problems because smoking causes deterioration of the blood vessels. A tissue expander implant procedure is often avoided for women with prior irradiation because the irradiated tissue does not expand well. The TRAM flap is preferred, since it will bring fresh tissue that is better able to heal than irradiated tissue. Women who have abdominal scars or who lack enough abdominal fat are not candidates for the surgery.

FREE FLAP

This procedure is sometimes called a free TRAM because an island of fat and skin is removed from the abdomen. However, rather than leaving a pedicle attached to its normal blood supply, the entire island is cut "free" and stitched in place over the mastectomy wound. A surgeon who specializes in microsurgery attaches the blood vessels supplying the flap to those in the chest wall. Because it's not necessary to remove as much muscle from the abdomen, the side effects of the TRAM muscle removal, including abdominal hernia, usually do not occur.

GLUTEUS FLAP

A free flap graft can also be made from the soft tissue, the skin, and the large (gluteus) muscle of the buttock. The free flap graft is typically performed when other options are not possible. It may cause hip problems, the sciatic nerve may become injured (causing leg pain, numbness, and weakness), and it is technically more difficult to accomplish than the free TRAM procedure.

Autologous breast reconstruction is major surgery that can require several hours in the operating room. The immediate complications are those associated with any operation—infection,
formation of blood clots in the legs (which is why you will be encouraged to move about in bed after surgery and get out of bed
the next day), and accumulation of blood and/or fluid in the
breast or donor site, which must be drained.

Much more likely—though still not common—are complications in healing. If the blood supply is not adequate, the skin over
the reconstructed breast may not heal properly and will die, requiring another operation to replace it. Sometimes, too, fatty tissue degenerates and causes a thickening that feels similar to a
lump or tumor, which can be very frightening. The surgeon may
then take a biopsy of the thickened area, to check for cancer cells.
Fluid or blood may continue to accumulate and must be withdrawn through a needle. Alternately, the surgeon may insert a
drain that allows the liquid to exit the body.

Nipple–Areola Reconstruction

To give the breast a realistic appearance, many women choose
to have the nipple and surrounding areola reconstructed also.
Several techniques can accomplish this; most often, tissue from
heavier skin in the upper inner thigh area is used. (Labial tissue is
not used.) Some tissue from just under the skin can create nipple
projection. The areola can be tattooed with a flesh-colored pig-
ment, but this refinement procedure is most often done only
after the reconstructed breast has healed completely.

Chapter 8

Radiation Therapy

Almost every plan for breast-conserving treatment (BCT) involves radiation therapy (RT). The treatment is local or regional rather than systemic; the goal is to have the radiation destroy cancer cells in a selected area. In the breast, "local" means the breast tissue and the muscle beneath the breast; "regional" includes the nearby axillary lymph nodes. Radiation therapy typically follows a lumpectomy, to destroy any undetected stray cancer cells in the breast and thereby prevent cancer recurrence. Studies indicate that RT can reduce local recurrence of breast cancer to less than 10 percent. After a mastectomy, if cancer recurs in the chest wall and skin, RT can control the disease in 50 percent of the women who have it. However, RT is not used immediately after mastectomy unless there is some reason to suspect cancer cells are present in the surgical area—for example, the tumor is larger than 5 centimeters, or cancer is found in several lymph nodes. When cancer cells cannot be removed by mastectomy, RT takes an active role in controlling their spread. In the past, RT was used to shrink a large tumor, making it easier to remove surgically; currently, this reduction in size is accomplished with preoperative chemotherapy.

THE RADIATION THERAPY TEAM

The science of radiation therapy is highly technical, and everyone involved in its use requires special training. The physician who designs your RT, cares for you during treatment, and monitors your recovery must have three or four years of training in radiology and cancer treatment and, after passing several examinations, earns certification by the American Board of Radiologists. This specialist, called a *radiation oncologist*, is usually recommended by a surgeon. When you are making your initial treatment decisions, you will probably consult with a radiation oncologist to learn what therapy, if any, is recommended.

During the actual treatment sessions, you will be cared for by *radiation technologists* who have special training in delivering to the appropriate site the exact dose of radiation ordered by your radiation oncologist. A *radiation therapist* keeps a detailed record of each treatment and notes your responses. *Radiation nurses*, registered nurses with special training in RT, are involved in delivering your treatment and helping you cope with the treatment itself and any side effects. The radiation oncologist might examine you once a week during treatment.

SELECTIVE DESTRUCTION

Various methods have been devised to deliver just enough radiation to damage the DNA of cancer cells, but not so much that many healthy cells are injured. In fact, modern techniques are so precise that minimal harm is done to the skin as the radiation beam passes through it, and there is little scattering of radiation to surrounding areas, such as the lungs and heart.

The Basics of Therapy

The type of radiation machine used will depend on the radiation oncologist's prescription. A combination of a cobalt and linear accelerator machine is most typical for the first course of treatment. The radiation is delivered in doses measured in rads (*radiation absorbed dose*). Another, more modern term often used is gray (Gy); 100 rads equals 1 gray. A typical dose following removal of a small breast cancer is 4,600 to 5,000 rads to the whole breast, and 1,200 to 1,600 rads to boost the area surrounding the lumpectomy site.

Preparing for Treatment

About four weeks after surgery, when healing is well under way, RT begins. If chemotherapy is prescribed, RT is usually delayed until the chemotherapy is finished. On your first postoperative visit to the radiation oncologist, the area to be irradiated is carefully measured. The size and location of the area to be treated are determined, and the precise angles at which that spot will be targeted are assessed. To accomplish this assessment, the radiation team uses a computerized device called a simulator. It is similar in appearance to the machine that will actually deliver the radiation dose during your subsequent visits.

In making the necessary measurements, the radiation oncologist will review the pathologist's report and all X-rays, including your pre- and postoperative mammograms. Small metal clips that were placed in the breast during surgery will be noted on the postoperative mammogram.

When all the calculations are made, the radiation therapist will make markings on your breasts and chest, around your collarbone, and/or under the arm on the surgery side, to indicate the exact areas to be irradiated. Sometimes, these marks are permanent. The technician also prepares a plaster mold that will fit around the back of your upper body. When you lie in the mold, it will hold you in the same position for each treatment. Because it includes measuring and marking your body, and fashioning a mold, this visit is quite time-consuming. Be prepared to spend about three or more hours at the radiation therapy center. The simulation visit also takes about two to three hours. Subsequent treatment visits are much shorter.

Before your treatment begins, you will be given instructions on how to prepare for the therapy, and what precautions you need to take. For instance, you cannot use deodorant, perfume, talcum powder, or deodorizing body soaps during the entire time you are receiving radiation therapy. These products contain certain ingredients, such as aluminum, that can interfere with radiation. Mild, fragrance-free soap is fine. Cornstarch or a solid deodorant crystal is permitted if you must use a deodorant. If you want to use any lotion or cream for dry skin, check the ingredients with the radiation oncologist to be certain the lotion will not cause problems. You will also be cautioned to avoid sun exposure during treatment.

In most hospitals and cancer treatment centers, you will be asked to sign an informed consent document similar to the one

My husband was fabulous. He was my caretaker. He would answer the phone. He would talk to people for me. We just went into hermit mode for four or five months. He would say to friends, "I'm sorry you haven't heard from us, but we've been in this tunnel. We don't know what anyone else is doing. We're just getting through what we're doing." He was amazing.

—J.C.

you signed before your biopsy and/or surgery. Typically, it states that you understand what is involved in the treatment.

Weekly Treatments

Most radiation oncologists prescribe five treatments a week, usually on consecutive days, for five or six weeks. This segment of treatment is sometimes followed by a series of boost sessions that may take five to ten days.

The actual treatment sessions are brief—thirty seconds or so—and you will soon become familiar with the routine. You undress from the waist up, remove any jewelry from around your neck, and cover yourself with a hospital gown or sheet. You then lie face up on an adjustable table. The arm on the side to be irradiated is usually placed behind your head. Only rarely are other placements used. The technician helps you into position on your plaster mold, which is kept in the radiation oncology facility. Finally, the radiation device is positioned over you so that it will target only the marked area. Your abdomen may be protected with a lead apron.

During the actual thirty-second treatment, the technician will be in an adjoining room, observing you through a window or on a video screen. An intercom allows you to be heard if you need any assistance.

The quick sequence of radiation emissions from different angles is silent, and there is no pain, nor are there any immediate aftereffects. The most uncomfortable part is keeping still and, sometimes, being chilled because your chest is exposed.

Women who work near a radiation therapy center are often able to schedule visits before work or during their lunch time, and they return to their jobs immediately afterward. Unfortunately, not all women are in such close proximity to a radiation center; for them, the daily treatments may be quite inconvenient and stress-provoking.

You may want someone to accompany you on your first visit or until you feel comfortable with the procedure, but assistance to and from the sessions should not be necessary.

After the third week of RT, your chest may become red and somewhat sensitive—some women describe a feeling similar to a mild sunburn, and some say the area itches and feels warm. Although this side effect is uncomfortable, it is not usually serious. However, a woman with large breasts who has had a lumpectomy may have to cope with more serious skin problems, such as peeling, blistering, soreness, and moistness under the fold of her breast.

During treatment, you must always cover the area if you are going into the sun, and never use heat or cold packs on this delicate skin. After treatment, you will want to protect the skin with a sunscreen or complete sun block. Because there may be some swelling or soreness during the treatment period, a loose-fitting camisole or a soft undershirt is more comfortable to wear than a bra. When the treatment and healing are complete, your radiation therapist and surgeon will let you know whether you can shave or use a depilatory cream or wax under the arm. This is usually not a problem.

In the last week or two of therapy, you may tire easily, and you may have to take time off from a busy schedule to rest. Tiredness, then, is to be expected, but debilitating fatigue is unusual. If you feel exhausted, tell your doctor. Blood tests are done at weekly intervals to ensure that you have a healthy *blood count*—an adequate number of red and white blood cells and platelets—especially if radiation follows chemotherapy.

If you have had a lumpectomy, you may notice that the irradiated breast becomes a bit firmer after RT. The skin may darken temporarily—perhaps for as long as a year—as it does with a sun-tan, and the nipple may become dry and sore. If you have had a mastectomy or lumpectomy, you may notice some soreness or stiffness in the chest muscle, and the area surrounding the incision may become thicker and firm. Axillary radiation therapy can also cause swelling of the arm or *lymphedema*, which requires special care (see pages 105–106).

It is unusual for women who receive RT to experience serious lasting side effects. Hair does not regrow under the arm in an area that has been irradiated, and the sweat glands may fail to regain their function—sometimes, permanently. Serious side effects cause problems for less than 1 percent of women treated with radiation. These complications include damage to the heart and ribs, and permanent damage to the soft tissue. Very rarely does the radiation cause a new cancer to form; when it does occur, decades have usually passed since treatment for the original cancer. The youngest women are most susceptible to this rare radiation effect, and since the incidence of new cancers begins after 15 years or so, they should be warned of their risk.

Chapter 9

Chemotherapy

Several decades ago, cancer specialists became aware that by the time a tumor was diagnosed as malignant, cancer cells may have spread to distant organs, even when no abnormalities were detected by a physical exam, X-rays, or any other tests. Because these *micrometastases* cannot be located and removed by surgery, and there is no way to know for certain that they exist, doctors rely on a *systemic* treatment: they treat the whole body to obliterate the malignant cells. Systemic treatment is usually called *adjuvant therapy* when it follows surgery and *neoadjuvant therapy* when it precedes surgery.

The first systemic treatment was a kind of antihormone therapy. Because female hormones can sometimes encourage breast cancer growth, doctors reasoned that curtailing the hormone supply—by removing a woman's ovaries or suppressing their activity with radiation therapy—would make cancer cells reproduce more slowly. In some women, particularly those who have not gone through menopause, this approach is still used. Then, in the 1940s, drugs that acted directly on the cancer cells were developed, and a new method called *chemotherapy* was introduced. Large studies of these drugs began in the 1950s; by the 1970s, chemotherapy was in widespread use.

Since that time, thousands of studies have been completed throughout the world to determine which drugs, used alone or in various combinations, are most likely to destroy malignant cells and prevent cancer from returning in the same site or in some other part of the body. Certain drug combinations are known to reduce the risk of breast cancer recurrence by at least one third. Newer drug combinations may be even more effective. Researchers continue to study different combinations of drugs and dosages, and alternate timing and intervals of treatment, in the hope of improving those statistics and developing new chemotherapy drugs that might offer better control of cancer, and possibly even a cure, with fewer side effects during and after treatment.

Like radiation, chemotherapy can be used to shrink large tumors. Studies are in progress to evaluate the use of *preoperative chemotherapy* or neoadjuvant treatment—chemotherapy before surgery—to destroy as many cancer cells as possible and thus shrink a large tumor before removing it.

Unless the cancer is detected very early and/or it is small and slow-growing, a surgeon will usually combine several treatments: surgery to remove the tumor (local control); radiation therapy to destroy any cancer cells remaining in the breast tissue (local control); surgery or radiation treatment of lymph nodes (regional control) plus chemotherapy (systemic control). Chemotherapy and radiation therapy are used together in various ways. One form of therapy may precede the other, or they may be given at the same time or alternated with each other. Thus far, there is little evidence to support one method of combining radiation and chemotherapy rather than another. Because systemic control is more important than local control, chemotherapy is often completed before radiation therapy begins.

If your breast surgeon or primary care physician wonders whether you might benefit from chemotherapy, he or she will refer you to a *medical oncologist,* a physician who is first trained in internal medicine and then board-certified in oncology, and who specializes in treating cancer medically—that is, with drugs—and managing the immediate and long-term side effects of chemotherapy. In many instances, the medical oncologist will become your primary physician, managing all aspects of your care after surgery.

When a medical oncologist recommends chemotherapy, it is advisable, for several reasons, to get a second opinion. You want to be certain that you are getting up-to-date advice, and you need to evaluate specific drug programs, which have different dosages and side effects. Also, opinions vary as to the best treatment in some situations—if, for instance, you have not yet gone through menopause or you have no cancer in your lymph nodes. By comparing recommendations, you will feel more confident about the treatment you finally choose. Cancer experts recommend consulting a medical oncologist even if your surgeon does not suggest chemotherapy.

HOW CHEMOTHERAPY WORKS

The main purpose of chemotherapy is to reach cancer cells through the bloodstream and kill them. Several types or classes of agents destroy cancer cells in various ways. Some cause permanent damage to a part of the cell that is involved with cell division, so the cell cannot reproduce itself. When the cell dies, there are no daughter cells to take its place. Other drugs work on other parts of the cellular growth and duplication systems. Combinations of drugs, therefore, are more effective than single drugs for control of most types of cancer. Cancer cells are dividing more rapidly than normal cells and are imperfect to begin with, so they are most vulnerable to any of these agents. However, because anticancer drugs are circulating in your bloodstream, they affect

other rapidly dividing cells—such as those in the scalp hair follicles, in the bone marrow, and in mucous membranes of the
mouth, vagina, intestines, and other organs. For normal cells, the
damage is temporary, but until healthy cells replace the injured
ones, unpleasant side effects occur.

Corticosteroids such as Prednisone affect the biological environment surrounding the cancer cells and inhibit their growth.
Corticosteroids were commonly given in the past because they
had this slight anticancer activity and they also helped to create a
feeling of well-being and to counter the side effects of chemotherapy, such as nausea. However, corticosteroid use is no longer so
common. Technically, any drugs used in cancer treatment are
usually labeled chemotherapy. However, in this discussion, antiestrogen drugs will be identified as hormone therapy.

Commonly Used Drug Combinations

Research has shown that the most effective chemotherapy for
breast cancer is a combination of drugs, each of which works in a
slightly different way. In the past, the most common treatment
combination for early-stage breast cancer was cyclophosphamide
(Cytoxan*), methotrexate, and 5-fluorouracil (5-FU), a combination commonly referred to as CMF. In different situations, other
drug combinations are recommended: CA, for cyclophosphamide
plus doxorubicin (or Adriamycin*), or CAF, for cyclophosphamide, doxorubicin (Adriamycin), and 5-fluorouracil. Although
doxorubicin is an especially powerful drug with many side effects,
its use for early-stage breast cancer is increasing. Recent studies
have found paclitaxel (Taxol), especially in combination with
other drugs such as cyclophosphamide and doxorubicin to be very

---

* Brand names: Cytoxan—Bristol-Myers Squibb; Adriamycin—Pharmacia and Upjohn.

effective. Some oncologist recommend drug combinations containing paclitaxel as initial treatment. Paclitaxel and a related drug, docetaxel (Taxotere*) are also useful treating women whose breast cancer recurred after treatment with other drugs.

Oncologists typically prescribe anticancer drugs in cycles, over a period of several months. For example, the standard program of CMF consists of eight cycles in which an intravenous (IV) injection is given once every three weeks. The drugs are spaced at regular intervals to allow their particular effect on the healthy cells to disappear before another dose of chemotherapy is given. Cyclophosphamide may also be taken in pill form every day, but the other drugs are given by injection.

Treatments given by injection or intravenously require that you go to the oncologist's office or the cancer care center at a hospital or clinic. The specific intervals between treatments are determined by the nature of the particular drugs prescribed and the predicted recovery of your normal cells. You will have periodic blood tests during the course of your chemotherapy, to be sure the drugs aren't damaging too many blood cells and to monitor your general health.

Chemotherapy can produce remission in women with metastatic breast cancer, but it is very important to discuss with the oncologist your prognosis or the outlook for your survival, and how the side effects may affect your quality of life.

In rare instances, your doctor may suggest *continuous infusion chemotherapy.* This slow and continuous delivery of minute quantities of a drug into the bloodstream allows you to receive doses of chemotherapy that would not be tolerated if given at one time. A tiny plastic catheter, smaller than a blood vessel, is inserted into a major vein and secured in place. The infusion may be done in a chemotherapy center or a hospital, but some types

* Brand name: Taxol—Bristol-Myers Squibb.

of continuous infusion equipment allow you to be mobile and go about your day-to-day activities. If it's necessary to receive the drug over twenty-four hours, the solution is carried with you in a purse, and the infusion tubing is camouflaged by your clothing.

Another option is *high-dose chemotherapy*—very high individual doses given over a brief period of time in one or two courses. Because this is a toxic therapy, you must be cared for in a hospital during the most difficult period of therapy, and your vital signs must be monitored. Because of the damage these doses of drugs do to your blood cells, you may be given other drugs to boost your blood cell production. In some cases, a bone marrow transplant (BMT) or peripheral blood stem cell transplant is necessary after the therapy, to restore your blood cells. More and more often, women have some of their own bone marrow or stem cells removed, stored, and reinfused (an autologous bone marrow transplant) after high-dose chemotherapy.

BMT is still an experimental therapy despite its increasing availability at large medical institutions throughout the country. Some insurance plans are now covering its cost. Because BMT has received so much positive attention in the media, its serious short-term risks (and some lasting, long-term ones) are often overlooked. High-dose chemotherapy followed by BMT has produced a complete remission in many women with breast cancer, but long-term studies of BMT's benefits and the chances of recurrence are still ongoing. BMT may be useful in some situations, and when the research is completed, those situations will be known. Overall, in breast cancer cases, there is no proof that high-dose chemotherapy with BMT prolongs life to a greater extent than moderate to high-dose chemotherapy not requiring BMT.

At any point during treatment, you can introduce new anti-cancer agents or treatments into your therapy by participating in a clinical trial.

Capecitabine (Xeloda*) is a promising new drug for breast cancer treatment. Unlike most chemotherapy drugs used in breast cancer treatment, capecitabine is taken as a pill. The drug itself does not kill the cancer cells directly. Once capecitabine enters the cancer cells, it is metabolized to 5-FU. The advantage of capecitabine, in addition to the convenience of its pill form, is that cancer cells actively convert it to 5-FU, but normal cells convert very little to 5-FU. As a result, capecitabine causes less damage to normal cells than an equivalent dose of intravenous 5-FU would. Preliminary studies indicate the new drug may help shrink about one-fourth of metastatic breast cancers that have not responded to standard chemotherapy.

Hormone Therapy

In the 1980s, a weapon called *hormone therapy* or *endocrine therapy* was added to the cancer treatment arsenal. In some women, especially those who have gone through menopause, breast cancer cells have receptors that respond to estrogen or progesterone. Antiestrogen drugs, such as tamoxifen, block these receptors. When deprived of the hormonal stimulation, the cancer cells replicate much more slowly or remain dormant. Eventually, the cells may die, although antihormone treatment cannot kill cells as some chemotherapy drugs do. In the past, hormone production was restricted only by removing the ovaries *(oophorectomy)* or irradiating them *(ovarian ablation)*. Those measures may still be used, though rarely, in women who have not gone through menopause and have advanced disease.

Studies show that tamoxifen, usually taken twice a day in pill form, is very effective in reducing the risk of breast cancer

---

* Brand name: Xeloda—Hoffman la Roche.

recurrence by as much as one-third. Researchers do not yet know the optimal time period for taking the drug, but it is usually prescribed for five years. After five years, tamoxifen is stopped because it has done as much as it can to affect the cancer cells, and possible side effects, such as endometrial cancer (cancer of the lining of the uterus; see Section III), must be considered.

Side Effects of Tamoxifen

Drugs that circulate in the bloodstream have the potential to cause side effects, and tamoxifen is no exception. It tends to cause symptoms similar to those of menopause, such as hot flashes, weight gain, and mood swings. Even though it is an antiestrogen drug, it produces some estrogenlike effects on certain organs. For instance, it stimulates the lining of the uterus, and 3 women in 1,000 taking 20 milligrams (mg) of tamoxifen a day eventually develop uterine cancer. The risk of endometrial cancer seems to increase with the duration of therapy beyond two years. While you are taking tamoxifen, your oncologist will caution you to report any abnormal vaginal bleeding, an early sign of uterine cancer. Regular gynecologic checkups, including an annual internal exam, are important as well.

About 1 percent of women who take tamoxifen develop *thrombophlebitis*, or clotting in the veins; your doctor will instruct you to report any new pain, redness, or swelling of the legs.

Those same estrogenlike effects also produce some benefits. For example, tamoxifen raises the amount of high-density lipoprotein (HDL)—the good form of cholesterol—in the bloodstream. In one study, there were 24 percent fewer deaths from cardiovascular disease among women on tamoxifen therapy than among those not on the drug. This is probably because the drug's long-term beneficial effects on cholesterol reduce the risk of atherosclerosis (hardening and blockage of the arteries). Tamoxifen also protects the bones and inhibits osteoporosis almost as well as estrogen taken after menopause.

The most important consideration in deciding whether or not you should receive adjuvant hormonal therapy with tamoxifen is the quantity of hormone receptors on your cancer cells. The greater the intensity of your hormone receptors' signals, the greater the likelihood that you will achieve excellent results with hormone therapy. On the other hand, having cancers with fewer or no detectable hormone receptors might be an argument for giving adjuvant chemotherapy alone, if indicated by the tumor's stage.

Tamoxifen is the most commonly used hormonal treatment, but there are others. Your doctor may suggest goserelin acetate or megestrol acetate. In addition to its use as adjuvant therapy of early breast cancer, hormonal therapy is also used to slow progression and relieve symptoms of advanced breast cancer.

WHO IS HELPED BY CHEMOTHERAPY?

A single micrometastasis spanning an eighth of an inch and cannot be detected by any scan or X-ray however it may be made up of more than a billion cancer cells. By destroying many of those cells—or preventing them from dividing—adjuvant therapy can increase the odds of a complete cure or, at least slow the course of the disease. Hundreds of adjuvant therapy studies have shown that adjuvant chemotherapy reduces the odds of death from breast cancer by at least one-fourth to one-third. In one important study in which the patients were followed for twenty years, the survival rate of women who had cancer in the lymph nodes and who were given adjuvant therapy was significantly better than the survival rate of those who did not get the systemic therapy. Because of this study's length, it showed once and for all that chemotherapy does not just delay recurrences but it actually has cured patients. Unfortunately, oncologists are unable to determine, before chemotherapy, who will benefit from it. But oncologists can make educated guesses that are fairly accurate. Here are some general guidelines for their recommendations.

At the top of the list for consideration of chemotherapy after breast cancer surgery is lymph node status. If breast cancer has spread to lymph nodes, chemotherapy is almost always indicated. When the lymph nodes seem to be free of cancer cells, adjuvant chemotherapy is still recommended: (1) if there is any reason to suspect that the cancer has already spread beyond the breast or (2) if other factors are present that put a woman at high risk for developing metastases. Your doctor will weigh the various characteristics of your particular cancer, your age, and your history, to determine whether you are at high risk (see Chapter 6). Most women with a breast cancer smaller than 1 centimeter (slightly less than a half-inch) and normal lymph nodes do not receive chemotherapy or tamoxifen.

Side Effects

Chemotherapy drugs are powerful and toxic, but there have been major improvements in the drugs themselves and in oncologists' knowledge of how to prescribe them. Furthermore, more drugs are available that can effectively relieve some side effects—such as nausea and vomiting—that were debilitating in the past.

HAIR LOSS

Without a doubt, hair loss is one of the most upsetting side effects of chemotherapy for women. For some women, the hair becomes noticeably thin and breaks easily, but some hair remains. For others, the scalp hair loss is total. The outcome depends a great deal on the drug given. Some women lose body hair also. Although it may help to know that your hair will grow back—and will sometimes be thicker, darker, and more curly than before—having your hair fall out in clumps is a serious injury to your self-image. In addition, hair loss is a public indication that you have an illness, and many women have a very difficult time letting others know that they are being treated for cancer. Some women never let anyone but their closest friends and family members know of their condition. This is a difficult path, but the effort to keep their disease more private is their method of coping.

Women who have been through the experience of hair loss can offer some suggestions on how to cope with it. Having your hair cut short before chemotherapy lessens the blow of having long hair come out in the shower or on your pillow. A short haircut helps you adjust to how you look with little or no hair. Women who wear wigs advise getting fitted before chemotherapy, and perhaps even buying the wig and having it styled ahead of time, so you don't have to go one day without this option. Participating in a support group of women with breast cancer who are undergoing or have had similar therapy can be a real help. The American Cancer Society's Look Good, Feel Better program (see Resources) can offer advice on selecting wigs. This program holds seminars to help women look their best and improve their self-image during treatment through the use of makeup, scarfs, hats, turbans, and wigs.

NAUSEA

This is a temporary side effect that tends to diminish between treatments. Nevertheless, nausea causes people to become anxious because they fear it will be debilitating. This is rarely the case, mainly because there are now several antinausea medications that prevent this side effect.

Some chemotherapy drugs cause nausea because of their effects on the brain rather than the gastrointestinal tract. The drugs increase the level of chemicals in the brain that are believed to stimulate an area called the *chemoreceptor trigger zone*. This same area is also stimulated by dizziness, which is why carnival rides that spin you around and upset your balance can make you sick. Anxiety also stimulates this area, which may explain why some people become nauseated just before their chemotherapy treatment begins.

How troubled you are by nausea depends a lot on the drugs in your treatment plan. Some cause only mild nausea or none at all; others could make nearly everyone sick, even to the point of vomiting. People react differently, too. Your doctor or nurse can tell you how the prescribed drugs make most women feel, but that does not mean you will have the same reaction.

If your chemotherapy does upset your stomach, taking antinausea medication before the treatment, and thereafter as prescribed for several doses, should control nausea. It also helps to alter your diet during the period when you tend to feel sick; eat smaller, more frequent meals of bland food, and avoid fried and spicy foods. Some people eat this way before receiving chemotherapy, too. Sucking on hard candy or mints can eliminate the unpleasant taste in the mouth that causes some people to feel nauseated. Snacking on dry saltines helps, too. If the smell of food cooking upsets your stomach, try to stay out of the kitchen when meals are being prepared, and eat your food at room temperature. Take sips of water frequently.

If vomiting is a problem, ask your doctor to prescribe your antinausea medication in suppository form. If vomiting occurs over a few days, watch for signs of dehydration: small amounts of dark urine (though some medications cause dark urine also), dizziness, and very dry mouth. Call your oncologist if you find you're unable to drink enough liquid.

For some people, relaxation exercises ease tension and relieve the anxiety that can make nausea even worse. Books and tapes are available to help you learn to relax.

SORE MOUTH

Some chemotherapy drugs cause the membranes lining the digestive tract, including the mouth, to become irritated. This temporary side effect can be relieved by avoiding spicy foods, very hot drinks, and acidic fruits and juices. Keeping your mouth clean, brushing your teeth with a soft toothbrush, and rinsing often with a mouthwash recommended by the oncologist all help relieve mouth soreness. Lip balms or a swipe of petroleum jelly can soothe dry lips.

FATIGUE

Feeling run down and lacking in energy is a side effect that people say seriously affects their quality of life during the period they are on chemotherapy. There are many reasons for the fatigue, from stress to the effects of the drugs themselves. If you have been nauseated, you may not have been eating or sleeping well, which adds to the fatigue. If your blood count is low and you are producing fewer red blood cells (which carry oxygen to your body tissues), you will feel tired and weak. Some causes of fatigue can be remedied, so it's important to report this side effect to your doctor rather than to assume that tiredness is inevitable.

WEIGHT GAIN

Several changes taking place during chemotherapy may contribute to weight gain. Many women become more sedentary during this stressful time. Some say they are actually hungrier, or they eat more high-calorie foods despite mild nausea. Experts do not believe that these explanations account for the average eight-pound weight gain that typically accompanies chemotherapy. Aerobic exercise can help control weight gain—and relieve mild nausea at the same time. Gaining weight could be a sign that you are retaining too much fluid. Report any sudden gains, or symptoms such as shortness of breath or swelling of your ankles or feet.

LOW BLOOD COUNTS

Chemotherapy causes the bone marrow to slow its production of red and white blood cells and platelets. Red cells carry oxygen to all the cells of the body, and white cells help fight infection. Platelets are important in blood clotting. Blood tests are taken routinely during therapy to monitor the blood count. If the numbers get too low, chemotherapy may be delayed until you build up a healthy quantity of blood cells.

A low white-cell count makes you vulnerable to infection. Having a low count seven to fourteen days after chemotherapy is not unusual, depending on the specific drugs. The white cells circulating in the bloodstream have expired, and fewer new ones have been manufactured in the bone marrow to replace them. This period is called the *nadir*. With a lower white-cell count, you have to be careful not be become infected with a cold virus, for example. It's especially important to eat a well-balanced diet and drink lots of fluids. Avoid large crowds if you can, and try to stay away from anyone with a cold or flu. Wash your hands often. Be alert for any signs of infection. If you have a fever, call your doctor. If you develop an infection, your oncologist will prescribe a powerful antibiotic. If your white blood cell count is dangerously low, new medications called growth factors can be given to stimulate your bone marrow to produce more blood cells. One example is filgrastim (Neupogen*), which stimulates production of white blood cells.

One particular type of bone marrow cells mature to become platelets, which are essential to plugging holes in damaged blood vessels. Bruising and bleeding gums are signs that your platelet count is low and should be reported to your doctor. Be careful not to cut yourself, and avoid risky contact sports or activities

---

* Brand name: Neupogen—Aargen.

until chemotherapy is complete. Brush your teeth with a soft toothbrush to prevent your gums from bleeding. If your platelet count drops too low, you may receive a platelet transfusion.

When your red blood cell count is low, you may be troubled by fatigue and dizziness. Your oncologist may prescribe iron supplements to help boost your blood supply, drugs that speed red blood cell production, or a red blood cell transfusion.

Long-Term Side Effects

Most of the unpleasant effects of chemotherapy dissipate after the treatment is finished, and normal cells replace the damaged ones. However, there may be lasting effects, depending on the drug(s) taken, the cumulative dose, and the individual.

MENOPAUSE

The older a woman is, the more likely that she will enter menopause during chemotherapy because of the drugs' effect on the ovaries. Hot flashes, insomnia, night sweats, and decreased vaginal lubrication are all symptoms that might now appear, exactly as they do when menopause occurs naturally.

In younger women, menstruation may become irregular and perhaps stop completely, though this is usually a temporary condition. Premature menopause or infertility does occur, however. If this is a possibility, your doctor will talk with you about it, or you should feel free to bring it up for discussion.

Currently one of the authors, Jeanne Petrek, is obtaining patients within six months of breast cancer diagnosis in order to study the determinants of premature menopause. The mail and phone research involves questionnaires and a menstrual cycle diary which will be analyzed in relation to specific chemotherapy drugs and dosages.

HEART PROBLEMS

Some drugs, especially doxorubicin (Adriamycin), can damage the muscle cells of the heart, sometimes leading to heart failure. According to studies of the drug's effects on the heart, the risk is greatest in those who receive the highest doses of doxorubicin, the elderly, and those with prior heart disease. A heart scan is usually performed before treatment, to evaluate and document cardiac function.

LEUKEMIA

Because chemotherapy affects the DNA of rapidly dividing cells, there is a chance that some normal cells—particularly those in the bone marrow—may be permanently damaged. When there is a mutation in the genes of developing blood cells, *leukemia*, a malignancy arising from white blood cells, may result. Some chemotherapy drugs are no longer used because of the risk of leukemia; those currently in use have a very low risk.

BREAST CANCER TREATMENT BY STAGE

Stage 0

The two types of Stage 0 breast cancer—ductal carcinoma in situ (DCIS) and lobular carcinoma in situ—(LCIS) are treated quite differently. No immediate treatment is recommended for most women with LCIS. But, having LCIS is a marker of increased risk for developing invasive cancer in either breast later on, so close followup is essential. A yearly mammogram and a clinical breast exam two or three times a year is suggested. These women may also wish to consider taking part in a clinical trial for breast cancer prevention. They may want to ask their doctors about other prevention strategies. A bilateral total or simple mastectomy may be an option for women with LCIS who have certain risk factors, such as strong family history, to prevent invasive cancer from developing.

Treatment of ductal carcinoma in situ (DCIS) depends on several factors. If the area of DCIS is small, a woman can usually choose between breast-conserving therapy (lumpectomy usually followed by radiation therapy) or simple mastectomy. If the area of DCIS is large or high grade, or if the breast contains several areas of DCIS, lumpectomy may not be possible, and mastectomy may be necessary. The five-year survival rate is 100 percent.

Stage I

One option is a lumpectomy with axillary lymph node dissection followed by radiation. Another option is modified radical mastectomy. If the tumor is less than 1 cm (about ½ inch) in diameter, adjuvant systemic therapy is not usually required. Some doctors recommend considering adjuvant therapy if the cancer has any unfavorable prognostic features (high grade, high S-phase fraction, or estrogen receptor negative). If the tumor is larger, adjuvant chemotherapy or hormonal therapy, or both, may be recommended. The five year survival rate for Stage I breast cancer is about 98 percent.

Stage II

Surgery and radiation therapy options for Stage I and Stage II tumors are similar, except that in Stage II, radiation therapy may be considered after mastectomy if the tumor is large or has spread to many lymph nodes. Adjuvant chemotherapy and/or hormonal therapy is usually recommended. If there are a lot of positive nodes (usually 10 or more) and the woman is in excellent health, she may choose to take part in a clinical trial of high-dose chemotherapy with stem cell transplantation. The five year survival rate for women with Stage IIA and IIB cancers are about 88 percent and 76 percent respectively.

Adjuvant Therapy for Stage I and Stage II Breast Cancer

Adjuvant chemotherapy and/or hormonal therapy may be chosen, based on the tumor's size, spread to lymph nodes, and prognostic features. Hormone therapy is not likely to be effective for women with estrogen receptor negative tumors, who usually receive chemotherapy only as their adjuvant therapy.

Postmenopausal women with estrogen receptor positive tumors often receive hormonal therapy with tamoxifen as their only adjuvant therapy. Some may also be treated with adjuvant chemotherapy.

Premenopausal women usually receive adjuvant chemotherapy. Until recently many premenopausal women with Stage I or Stage II breast cancer did not receive tamoxifen, but recent studies have shown that they are helped by the drug, which reduces their risk of recurrence and improves survival rates.

Stage III

This stage is divided into two parts, IIIA and IIIB. Smaller Stage IIIA breast cancers may be removed by modified radical mastectomy and lumpectomy may sometimes be an option. Surgery is usually followed by radiation therapy and adjuvant systemic therapy. Larger Stage IIIA cancers may be treated with *neoadjuvant* chemotherapy, with or without hormonal therapy, followed by a modified radical mastectomy. A lumpectomy may be an option, but this approach is considered somewhat experimental. In either case, surgery is usually followed by radiation therapy and more systemic therapy (chemotherapy, with or without hormonal therapy).

For Stage IIIB, the treatment is neoadjuvant chemotherapy, with or without hormonal therapy, followed by lumpectomy or radical mastectomy, and then sometimes more chemotherapy. The goal of neoadjuvant therapy in Stage III breast cancer is to shrink the tumor so it can be removed more completely or easily by surgery. After surgery, radiation therapy and more chemotherapy, with or without hormonal therapy, is given. Patients with Stage IIIB cancer may consider clinical trials of high-dose chemotherapy with stem cell transplantation. The five-year survival rate for Stages IIIA and IIIB are about 56 percent and 49 percent, respectively.

Stage IV

Chemotherapy and/or hormonal therapy are the main options. Radiation and/or surgery may also be used to provide relief of certain symptoms. Patients in otherwise good health are encouraged to take part in clinical trials of high-dose chemotherapy or other promising but unproven treatments. The five-year survival rate is approximately 16 percent.

Part II
The Cervix

Chapter 10

The Healthy Cervix

The cervix doesn't secrete hormones or regulate reproduction, yet it serves a vital function in conception and pregnancy. The mucus secreted by glands in the cervix allows sperm to pass into the uterus; the tightly closed cervix holds the developing fetus in the uterus during pregnancy. In labor, the walls of the cervix become thin, and the tiny opening at its center dilates, allowing the baby to enter the vagina or *birth canal*. The central opening is so narrow that, under normal conditions, little can penetrate it, yet menstrual blood and tissue can easily flow from the uterus into the vagina. However, the cervix is not impenetrable. It is now known that bacteria and viruses can pass through the cervical opening and enter the uterus and fallopian tubes.

WHAT IS THE CERVIX?

Cervix is the Latin word for neck; the cervix is the narrow neck of the uterus that projects into the upper third of the vagina. The cervix is about one inch long. The opening in the center, called the *cervical canal*, is the entry point to the hollow body of the uterus (the *uterine corpus*). In a woman who has not had children, the opening, or *os*, is about the size of a pencil point. In a woman who has given birth, it looks like the mouth of a fish.

There is a slight narrowing where the upper cervix (endo-cervix) meets the lower cervix (ectocervix). The endocervix joins the body of the uterus; the ectocervix projects into the vagina. The cervix is supplied with blood through branches of the uterine artery and other arteries that extend upward from the vagina. Veins carry oxygen-depleted blood away from the cervix along a parallel pathway. A network of lymphatic vessels carries lymph from the cervix to the pelvic lymph nodes (Figure 10.1).

Although the uterus, of which the cervix is a part, is a muscular organ, the cervix itself consists of more connective tissue. It

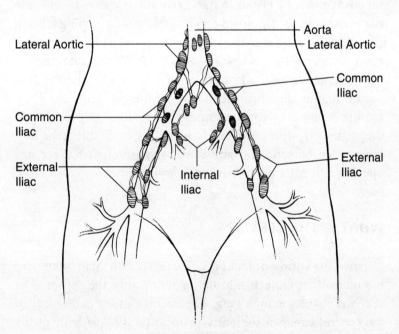

Figure 10.1: Major lymph nodes of the pelvis.

has been said that if you were to touch your cervix with your fingertip, it would feel like the tip of your nose.

The endocervix is lined with cylindrical epithelial cells and contains many mucus-producing glands. This mucus helps keep infectious organisms out, but it is not a complete barrier. As ovulation nears, the consistency of the mucus thins, enabling sperm to enter through the canal into the uterus.

The ectocervix is lined with flat epithelial cells called squamous cells. The area where the upper and lower portions of the cervix meet is known as the *transformation zone*. During the reproductive years, this zone is lower in the cervix than later in life. After menopause, for example, this area withdraws high into the cervix. The transformation zone is the area where most cervical cancers begin, so health care professionals are very interested in assuring that Pap test specimens include cells from this zone.

SCREENING

Over fifty years ago, Dr. George Papanicolaou devised a method for examining under a microscope the cells shed from the outermost layer of the cervix. This test, called a Papanicolaou or *Pap test* or *Pap smear,* is now used routinely to detect abnormalities on the cervix. There is a common misconception that a Pap test diagnoses all cancer of the reproductive tract. It is *not* a sensitive screening test for cancers of the ovaries, fallopian tubes, or the body of the uterus.

The Pap test is a screening tool. Although the laboratory results may strongly indicate that cancer is present, it is necessary for the doctor to retrieve, via a *biopsy,* a sample of tissue from the cervix for examination under a microscope. Only then can a diagnosis be definitive. A Pap test can identify cellular changes that are precancerous, and it can indicate changes that are typically associated with infection by various organisms, including sexually transmitted diseases such as human papilloma virus (HPV) and herpes. It can also detect infection with yeast and trichomonas. A sample of cells obtained at the same time as the Pap smear can be tested for chlamydia.

No randomized clinical trials have been done to prove that examination of cells from the cervix saves lives, but the dramatic and steady decrease in the incidence of cervical cancer and the 70 percent decline in deaths from the disease since the Pap test was made widely available are proof of its effectiveness as a screening test.

This success notwithstanding, the Pap test is a topic of much concern. The current debate focuses on how often the Pap test is needed, who should have it, and how to ensure accurate results.

Who Needs a Pap Test?

The American Cancer Society recommends an annual Pap test and a pelvic examination for all women over age eighteen and for younger women who are sexually active. After three years—and three consecutive, satisfactory negative Pap tests—a woman and her health care provider can determine how often to repeat the test, depending on the woman's physical condition, sexual habits, and other risk factors. (Women over age forty should have an annual pelvic examination even when they don't have a Pap test.)

Older women, who tend not to have pelvic examinations as often as younger women, sometimes fail to have Pap smears at all, and their doctors sometimes fail to encourage them to have the test. Screening for changes in the cells of the cervix is important throughout life. Cancer of the cervix may take years to develop, and women who have had normal Pap smears in their middle years may suddenly have an abnormal result long after menopause. Statistics indicate that the incidence of and the mortality rate from cervical cancer increase with age. Invasive cervical cancer occurs most often in women between the ages of forty and sixty.

It might seem that a woman who has had a *total hysterectomy* (removal of the uterus and cervix) for a benign condition no longer needs a regular Pap test because she no longer has a cervix, but some experts say that she should have a Pap test of the cells of the vagina every three to five years. Those who have had a *partial or subtotal hysterectomy* (removal of the body of the uterus but not the cervix) should follow the same screening guidelines as other women their age. A woman who has had a hysterectomy because of cancer should have a regular Pap test of the vagina every six months following the surgery for a minimum of two years, and annually thereafter.

How the Pap Test Is Done

The Pap test is simple, quick, and relatively painless. The test may be done by various health care providers—a physician, a nurse practitioner, or a physician's assistant—but the main criterion is that the person doing the test has had adequate training in how to correctly obtain the smear. A very specific technique must be followed for accurate results.

To perform the test, the health care provider will use a metal or plastic speculum to spread the walls of the vagina and will visually examine the surface of the cervix. This is not a painful procedure, but there may be some discomfort. Then he or she swipes the ectocervix with a thin wooden or plastic spatula. A cotton swab or a cytobrush is used to sample cells from the endocervix and the transformation zone (Figure 10.2).

The sample is wiped across a laboratory slide, and a special fixative spray or solution is applied to it. The sample is sent to a laboratory for microscopic examination by a technologist who has

Preparing for a Pap Test

Certain activities and conditions should be avoided before a Pap test, to make sure the results are accurate. The following is a list of dos and don'ts:

- Do not douche for at least twenty-four hours before the test. (Some authorities recommend avoiding douching for two to three days before the test.)
- Do not use any kind of vaginal cream, foam, or suppository for at least twenty-four hours before the test.
- Do not have sexual intercourse for twenty-four hours before the test.
- Do not have the test while you are menstruating. The best time for a Pap test is at least five days after menstruation stops.

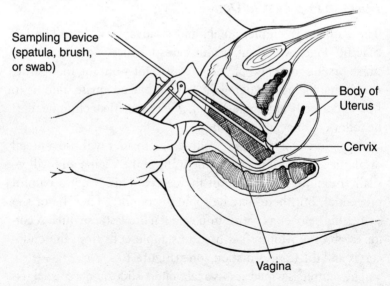

Figure 10.2: The Pap test.

special training in examining Pap smears (cytotechnologist). If abnormal cells are detected, a pathologist will examine the slide. (See the discussion of ThinPrep in the next section.)

How Accurate Is It?

The potential for a *false-negative* report—in which the Pap test result indicates there are no cancer cells present when there actually are—has received a great deal of attention in recent years. There have been problems with laboratories' failure to detect cancer cells, but a false-negative Pap test can also be the result of the health care provider's error in retrieving the cell sample or his or her failure to apply the fixative promptly. Pap test samples that do not include cells from the transformation zone, the area where most cervical cancers develop, are more likely to have false negative results. Traditionally a cotton swab has been used to sample this area, but many doctors prefer other sampling devices such as the cytobrush that are more effective in obtaining transformation zone cells. Fortunately, cervical cancer usually grows so slowly that if a woman has a Pap smear every year, an abnormality that is missed one year is likely to be detected in the next test, with no ill effect from the year-long delay.

A false positive result means that the woman's cervix is normal, but the test indicated that cancer or a precancerous condition was present. Then results can cause great anxiety and lead to unnecessary tests. But, treatment is not started until a Pap test result is confirmed by biopsy, so the negative consequences of a false positive result are limited. False negative results on the other hand can have very serious consequences if a rapidly spreading cancer is missed.

In the past ten years, a great deal of attention has been given to the problem of laboratory errors in interpreting Pap smear results. In 1988, Congress passed the Clinical Laboratory Improvement Act (CLIA), and it went into effect in 1992. According to this act, laboratories must follow certain regulations that are intended to ensure the accuracy of tests.

In recent years, the FDA has approved three adjunctive methods aimed at improving the accuracy of the Pap test.

One approach to improving Pap test accuracy is to change how cells are placed on the microscope slide. Usually, the sample is smeared directly onto the slide. This means that cells are sometimes piled up on each other, and some cells at the bottom of the pile may not be clearly seen. Also, infections of the cervix or vagina may cause inflammatory cells, increased mucus, yeast cells, or bacteria that hide the cervical cells. Another problem with direct smears is that the cells may become distorted by drying out, if the fixative solution is not added promptly, making them difficult to examine accurately. A new method can remove some of the mucus, bacteria, yeast, and inflammatory cells in a sample and can spread the cervical cells more evenly on the slide. This new method, called the *ThinPrep**, also prevents distortion of the cells due to delayed fixation. Instead of directly placing the sample on a slide, it is immediately placed into a special preservative solution. A special instrument in the laboratory then removes cells from the solution and places them on a glass microscope slide. Recent studies indicate that this new method can slightly improve detection of cancers, significantly improve detection of early precancers, and reduce the number of tests that need to be repeated. Whether or not this method has a significant impact on preventing cancer and whether it is the best approach to improving the Pap test needs to be studied

---

* Brand name: ThinPrep—Cytyc Corp.

further. This method is not used by most laboratories and is more expensive than a usual Pap test.

Another approach to Pap test improvement is the use of computerized instruments that can recognize abnormal cells in Pap smears. Two instruments, the *PAPNET** and the *AutoPap**, are currently approved by the United States Food and Drug Administration (FDA) for double-checking samples after examination by technologists. The instruments can be used to retest Pap smear samples that were interpreted as normal by technologists. The AutoPap is also approved by the FDA for initial screening of Pap smears, instead of screening by a technologist. A technologist would still examine all smears identified as abnormal by the AutoPap, however. These instruments can find abnormal cells that are sometimes missed by the technologists. But, most of the abnormalities found in this way are relatively early ones, such as atypical squamous cells of undetermined significance (ASCUS). Many doctors are not convinced that finding more of these early abnormalities will have a significant impact on preventing invasive cervical cancers.

The current automated screening instruments have two disadvantages. One is that they sometimes identify samples as abnormal when the woman has a normal cervix. As a result, she may undergo an unnecessary colposcopy. The second disadvantage is their expense, which more than doubles the cost of the Pap test. Most laboratories do not use computerized screening instruments yet. Although there is some debate among doctors as to whether current instruments should be used for Pap testing, many agree that improvements in the near future will improve accuracy and lower cost, and that they will eventually become an important aid to Pap testing.

* Brand name: PAPNET—Neuromedical Systems, Inc.; AutoPap—NeoPath, Inc.

BETHESDA SYSTEM (TBS) CLASSIFICATIONS

Description	What It Means
Within normal limits	No signs of cancer or precancerous changes.
Benign cellular changes	Normal cells with changes related to infection or repair of minor damage.
Infection	Possible infection with herpes, yeast, trichomonas, or other microorganism.
Reactive and reparative changes	Signs of cell regeneration. This may be due to tissue injury caused by inflammation (infection), radiation, an intrauterine device, or certain hormonal changes.
Atypical squamous cells of undetermined significance (ASCUS)	Unable to tell whether the abnormality is due to tissue injury and repair or to a precancer.
Epithelial cell abnormalities	Potentially precancerous changes or cancer.
Low-grade squamous intraepithelial lesion (SIL)	Mildly abnormal cells, often with HPV infection. The cervix usually returns to normal without treatment but, in some women, the abnormal cells may later develop into cancer.
High-grade squamous intraepithelial lesion (SIL)	Cells have a greater degree of abnormality, and greater risk of developing into cancer than with low-grade SIL.
Squamous cell carcinoma	Cells are cancerous. This is a type of cancer that develops from the squamous cells of the ectocervix or transformation zone.
Atypical glandular cell of undetermined significance	Unable to determine whether the glandular cell abnormality is due to tissue injury and repair or to cancer.

Adenocarcinoma	Cells are cancerous. This type of cancer develops from the gland cells of the endocervix. It can also start in the endometrium, fallopian tube, or ovary.

What Does the Report Mean?

Depending on the degree of abnormality seen in the cells, the pathologist will classify it according to one of several different systems. For many years, laboratories used class numbers ranging from Class I (no abnormal cells) to Class V (malignant cells). In 1988, the Bethesda System (TBS) for Reporting Cervical-Vaginal Cytological Diagnoses was devised in order to have one uniform and specific language for describing the Pap test results. The Bethesda System is important because it reports whether the sample was adequate for an accurate assessment, and it provides a general categorization of the specimen, as noted in the box below. The classification was modified in 1991.

Low- and high-grade squamous cell abnormalities (SIL) may also be referred to as CIN (for cervical intraepithelial neoplasia) or dysplasia. CIN 1 is also called mild dysplasia or a low-grade SIL. CIN 2 is moderate dysplasia. CIN 3 is severe dysplasia or carcinoma in situ. Both CIN 2 and CIN 3 are included in the category of high-grade SIL.

In cases of high-grade SIL, the next step is clearly a diagnostic test such as colposcopy or biopsy or both. What to do with a low-grade SIL (mild dysplasia or CIN 1), however, is currently being debated. Some physicians recommend further diagnostic tests; others believe that because the low-grade abnormality often reverses itself, the Pap test should be repeated in a few months. It is important not to ignore these changes and to get follow-up care.

Chapter 11

Who Is at Risk?

The relationship between cancer of the cervix and the human papilloma virus (HPV) that causes genital warts is so strong that many experts consider cervical cancer a sexually transmitted disease (STD). After a woman is infected with HPV, over a period of months or years, the cells of her cervix may be transformed by the virus into abnormal, precancerous cells known as CIN, or *cervical intraepithelial neoplasia*. After a latency period varying from less than a year to decades, these cells may become malignant, if not treated in the precancer phase.

Beginning sexual activity at a young age (that is, before age seventeen), having multiple sex partners, having sexual relations with a man who has had multiple partners, and having unprotected sex all increase a woman's risk of encountering HPV and, subsequently, developing cervical cancer. Having sexual relations with a man whose previous partner had cancer of the cervix is also a risk factor. This does not mean that cancer cells are transmitted. The probable explanation involves transmission of a high risk HPV type. Women who have had one monogamous sexual partner are at low risk for cancer of the cervix. Using a barrier method of birth control, such as condoms or a diaphragm can also lower the risk because it helps protect the cervix against HPV transmission. However, a diaphragm does not protect against some other STDs, such as human immunodeficiency virus (HIV).

There are more than seventy different types of HPV, and over twenty types are known to affect the anus and genital tract. Of those twenty, some types are more likely than others to stimulate the growth of abnormal cells. Most genital warts are caused by HPV types 6 and 11, but these rarely cause cancer. However, there are high-risk HPV types (such as 16, 18, 33, and 45) that have been associated with genital or anal cancers in men and women.

A Pap smear can reveal changes in cervical cells that are caused by HPV infection, and special DNA tests can identify the type of virus present. At this time, though, HPV testing and typing are not routinely recommended. There is no cure for HPV infection, but the proliferation of infected cells can be destroyed, which prevents them from developing into cancer.

Although HPV infection is associated with 93 percent of all cases of cervical cancer, not all women with HPV develop the disease—nor do all women with the cancer have HPV. These facts lead many researchers to believe that other factors play a role. Perhaps the DNA in cervical cells is damaged in such a way that the cells no longer die and are shed but continue making abnormal copies of themselves. (This excessive proliferation of cells may become cervical cancer.)

Some researchers think that genital herpes virus is involved, but evidence for this theory is not conclusive. Studies have linked smoking to cervical cancer. Interestingly, women who have cervical cancer are at increased risk for developing lung cancer later. Researchers who examined the cervical mucus of smokers found that these women had much higher concentrations of nitrosamines—cancer-causing substances that come from tobacco smoke—in their mucus than nonsmokers. These chemicals are absorbed by the lungs and travel through the blood to all parts of the body. Recently, there have been reports linking cervical cancer with a sexual partner's smoking habits. Carcinogenic agents from cigarettes may be in a male partner's semen or may coat his fingers, which then contaminate the vagina during coital caressing. Another explanation is second-hand smoke from the partner's cigarettes. However, many of these studies have not tested for HPV nor controlled for it in their analysis.

In the past decade, researchers have been investigating nutritional risk factors. Women with cervical cancer have been found to have low levels of the vitamin A precursor, beta carotene, and of vitamin C and folic acid. This discovery has led some experts to recommend frequent screening of women who are malnourished. There is a relationship between low socioeconomic status and an increased incidence of cervical cancer, and, in part, that may be due to poor nutrition.

Some researchers think that the hormones in oral contraceptives may be a cofactor, with HPV, in causing cervical cancer. However, other factors may be involved. For example, when most studies of oral contraceptive users were done, women taking "the Pill" may have been more likely to have multiple sexual partners than were women who did not take it and did not use condoms or a diaphragm.

When a woman has an abnormal Pap test, her risk of cancer increases. According to one study, women treated for carcinoma in situ who continued to have abnormal Pap results were about twenty-four times more likely to develop invasive cervical cancer than those who had normal follow-up Pap test results.

Women who have suppressed immunity for any reason have a high risk of developing cancer of the cervix, and the risk for those infected with the human immunodeficiency virus (HIV) is especially high. In fact, cervical cancer is now considered to be an AIDS-related cancer.

Although the incidence of cervical cancer is low in women whose mothers took diethylstilbestrol (DES) during their pregnancy, these so-called "DES daughters" have an increased risk of developing a rare type of cervical cancer called clear cell adenocarcinoma.

Chapter 12

Precancerous Conditions

Although cancer of the cervix remains the second leading cause of death from cancer throughout the world, mortality rates in the United States have dropped sharply. The main reason for the decline in this country has been screening with the Pap test, which has become a routine aspect of women's health care. Abnormal conditions are discovered—and treated—early.

If you learn that your Pap test was abnormal, don't panic. Some doctors wrongly recommend immediately repeating the test; others point out that it may yield a false-negative result. Depending on the type of abnormality, your health care provider may want to repeat the test in three or four months, or he or she may recommend a colposcopy and possibly a biopsy. If there is an infection or inflammation of the cervix, the Pap test can be repeated after the condition has been treated.

FURTHER EVALUATION

To determine why a Pap test was abnormal and what your current situation is, several steps are possible. The examinations and techniques described below may be suggested to you by your physician.

Colposcopy

Often, a physician will rely on a technique called *colposcopy* to check for any visible *lesions*, an area of abnormal tissue, or a tumor. Colposcopy involves direct examination through a binocular-like instrument that magnifies the surface of the cervix six to thirty times. Your gynecologist may do this examination or may refer you to a gynecologic oncologist who specializes in colposcopy.

The procedure isn't painful, but it can be uncomfortable because you have to maintain the same position with a vaginal speculum in place for up to fifteen minutes. With the speculum holding the vaginal walls open, the cervix is washed with an acetic acid or vinegar solution that may sting slightly. The viewing colposcope does not actually touch your cervix but is placed close enough to the open speculum to allow your health care provider to directly view the cervix.

Cervicography

Because of the significant false-negative rate of Pap tests, some physicians follow a Pap smear with *cervicography*, a quick, simple, and painless procedure in which the surface of the cervix is photographed with a special camera called a *cerviscope*. The 35-millimeter photograph can then be enlarged and sent to an expert to be examined for abnormalities. Even though some gynecologists find cervicography quite useful, it is not a standard procedure and is still considered investigational.

Biopsy

If your physician detects any obviously abnormal areas, he or she will do a biopsy. The most common type is a *punch biopsy* or *directed biopsy* in which one or more small pieces of tissue are removed from abnormal-appearing areas of the cervix. *Endocervical curettage (ECC)*, a scraping of small tissue fragments from the endocervical canal, may also be done at this time. The cervix is not dilated, but the procedure may be somewhat painful for a brief moment. Some women describe it as a mild cramping similar to a menstrual period. Your doctor may prescribe a nonnarcotic pain reliever or a local anesthetic beforehand. Endocervical curettage is not done on pregnant women.

There may be some bleeding following a biopsy and/or endocervical curettage. And for up to two weeks after either procedure, women are usually instructed to avoid douching, intercourse, and using tampons, in order to prevent infection while the area heals.

When a biopsy has confirmed that a lesion is precancerous, there are several ways to destroy the abnormal cells. The lesion can be vaporized with a laser, killed by freezing with liquid

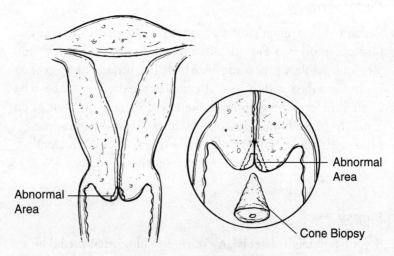

Figure 12.1: Cone biopsy.

nitrogen or carbon dioxide (cryosurgery), or by burning (cauterization), or gradually sloughed away with a tissue-destroying cream such as 5-FU. These methods are called *ablative* procedures. The lesion can also be removed by surgical procedures known as cone biopsy and LEEP.

Depending on the location and severity of the lesion, any of these ablative or surgical procedures may be considered. If several procedures are suitable for your situation, your doctor is likely to recommend the one with which he or she has the most experience and is most appropriate to your situation.

CONE BIOPSY

A *cone biopsy* is the excision of a cone-shaped piece of tissue from the center of the cervix that includes the opening at its center (see Figure 12.1). A cone biopsy—also known as *cold knife biopsy* or *conization*—is a more complicated procedure than a directed or punch biopsy, and requires general anesthesia. It can be done on an outpatient basis. An overnight stay in the hospital is usually not required unless there is heavy bleeding or some other problem following the surgery.

For a few days after the procedure, there is usually a discharge and possibly some bleeding. To prevent infection, intercourse, douching, and use of vaginal tampons should be avoided for about four to six weeks, or until healing is complete.

A physician typically recommends a cone biopsy if one (or more) of these situations occurs:

1. If there is a discrepancy between the results of the punch biopsy and the Pap test.
2. If the lesion cannot be seen entirely by colposcopy, or the ECC is positive.
3. If the biopsy indicates microinvasive cancer.

Complications from this surgery are rare, but a very large cone biopsy can affect the cervical mucus and lead to fertility problems. Rarely does the cervix become incompetent—that is, dilating too early in pregnancy.

LOOP ELECTROSURGICAL EXCISION PROCEDURE (LEEP)

This relatively new biopsy technique may be used as an alternative to cone biopsy in most situations. It's simpler and less expensive than the standard cone biopsy method. In a single pass of a thin, electrified, wire loop over the cervix, the surgeon removes the abnormal transformation zone for further study under a microscope. Usually, a local anesthetic is sufficient to numb the cervix, and colposcopy is done prior to surgery so that the doctor can clearly see the area he or she wants to remove.

During the procedure, the electrified wire loop cuts tissue and coagulates severed blood vessels at the same time. Afterward, the doctor may apply a thin layer of a special blood-coagulating gel to the surface of the cervix.

Although LEEP, which is sometimes called simply loop biopsy, was designed to remove a lesion for further study, an entire area of intraepithelial neoplasia (CIN) may be excised, resulting in complete treatment as well.

A pathologist will examine the tissue under a microscope and will search the edges of the tissue removed by cone biopsy or LEEP to be certain no areas of CIN or invasive cancer are present. If these *margins* contain CIN or invasive cancer, the edges of the wound on the cervix is also likely to have areas of CIN or invasive cancer and additional surgery may be necessary. Discuss with your doctor how CIN with positive margins will be managed. If invasive cancer is found, additional surgery or radiation therapy will be necessary as discussed in the next chapter.

Chapter 13

When the Diagnosis Is Cancer

When cancer cells invade tissues beneath the surface or epithelial layer of the cervix, a woman has *invasive cancer*. Warning signs may include unusual vaginal bleeding or discharge, but unless the cancer is very advanced, there are rarely any symptoms. Invasive cancer may be identified by a Pap test and a biopsy. Sometimes, a Pap test detects a cervical intraepithelial neoplasia (CIN), and when the gynecologist does a colposcopy and biopsy, an invasive cancer is discovered. It's important to understand that cervical cancer is a preventable disease. If all women were regularly screened with a Pap test and had precancers treated appropriately, the disease could be eliminated almost entirely.

In most cases, it takes several years for carcinoma in situ—cancer cells in the uppermost layer of the cervix—to become invasive. But this sometimes happens within a year, which is why it is so important to have annual Pap tests and to treat any significant abnormalities without delay.

The depth of the invasion and the general extent of the disease—that is, whether it has spread to lymph nodes and other parts of the body—determine the cancer's *stage*. It's very important for your doctor to establish the stage of your disease and for you to understand exactly what it means. The treatments your doctors recommend are based on the stage that is diagnosed and, to a great extent, so is your prognosis. When you know both the stage of your cancer and your prognosis, you will be more prepared to participate in making decisions about your treatment. Other factors that will influence your choice of treatment include yo'ır age, your general health, and, if you are premenopausal, your desire to have children.

The various staging systems and their terminology can be confusing, so when your doctor discusses staging with you, be certain you understand what system he or she is using: the International Federation of Gynecology and Obstetrics (FIGO) system or the American Joint Committee on Cancer (AJCC) system. Most oncologists use the FIGO system for staging cervical cancer.

Both systems require a biopsy of the tumor, depending on the results of the biopsy and physical examination, various further tests may also be needed, such as X-rays of the chest and kidneys; *proctoscopy*, in which the anus and rectum are examined through a special viewing instrument called an *endoscope*; and *cystocopsy*, in which the bladder is inspected through an endoscope. Surgery to inspect the pelvic organs and selective biopsy of the lymph nodes may be performed to assess the extent of disease, but is not part of the staging procedure. These tests allow your physician to determine whether the cancer has spread, and if so, how extensive it is.

TYPES OF CERVICAL CANCER

The *type* describes the kind of cell or tissue in the cervix that the cancer is derived from. Ninety percent of cervical cancers are

STAGING OF CANCER OF THE CERVIX

FIGO Stage   *Description*

I Cervical cancer confined to uterus.

    IA Preclinical cervical cancer (visible only when magnified under a microscope).

        IA1 Preclinical cervical cancer with area of invasion less than 3 millimeters (about $\frac{1}{8}$ inch) deep and less than 7 millimeters (about $\frac{1}{3}$ inch) wide.

        IA2 Preclinical cervical cancer with area of invasion between 3 millimeters (mm) and 5 mm (about $\frac{1}{5}$ inch) deep. The width of the invasive cancer is less than 7 mm.

    IB Cervical cancer that can be seen without a microscope and/or is larger than a Stage IA2 cancer.

        IB1 A IB cancer that is no larger than 4 centimeters (about $1\frac{3}{5}$ inches).

        IB2 A IB cancer that is larger than 4 centimeters.

II Cervical cancer that has spread to the upper $\frac{2}{3}$ of the vagina and/or the tissues next to the cervix *(parametrial tissue)*, but has not spread to the wall of the pelvis.

    IIA A Stage II cervical cancer that involves part of the vagina but not as far as the lower third of the vagina.

    IIB A Stage II cervical cancer that has spread to the tissue next to the cervix *(parametrial tissue)*.

III Cervical cancer that has spread to the lower third of the vagina and/or to the pelvic wall and/or blocks urine flow from the kidney to the bladder causing kidney damage and accumulation of too much urine in the kidney.

    IIIA A Stage III cancer that has spread to the lower third of the vagina but not to the pelvic wall, and has not caused urine blockage or kidney damage.

    IIIB A Stage III cancer that extends to the pelvic wall, causes kidney damage and/or accumulation of too much urine in the kidney.

IV Cervical cancer to nearby organs such as the bladder or rectum, and/or has spread to distant organs.

    IVA A Stage IV cancer with spread to the inner lining *(mucosa)* of the bladder or rectum.

    IVB A Stage IV cancer with spread (metastasis) to distant organs.

squamous cell carcinomas that develop from squamous epithelial cells of the ectocervix and transformation zone. About 10 percent are adenocarcinomas that develop from endocervical glandular cells. In rare situations, adenosquamous and small cell carcinomas are found.

Chapter 14

Treatment

As in most cancers, treatment of cancer of the cervix depends primarily on the stage of the disease. The stage describes the size of the tumor, whether it extends into surrounding tissues and/or structures and whether it has spread to distant organs. Your age, your desire to have children, and your general health must be considered as well. For example, when a young woman has carcinoma in situ or very early cancer of the cervix, she may be a candidate for conization, a conservative treatment in which a cone-shaped piece of cervical tissue that contains the cancer is removed (see Figure 12.1). (Carcinoma in situ means that the cancer cells have not yet invaded the deeper tissues of the cervix but are found only in the lining.) If cancer cells are found at the edges of the cone biopsy, a hysterectomy may still be necessary, but this conservative approach (cone biopsy) is usually sufficient. A follow up endocervical curretage and colposcopy will usually be done three to four months after the cone biopsy to see if additional treatment is needed.

The procedure your physician prefers is often the one that you are encouraged to have. Doctors tend to be partial to one approach because they have more experience with that treatment. However, to better understand the risks and the benefits of all your options, it's often a good idea to get at least one other opinion.

TREATMENT OPTIONS

For the most part, cervical cancer is treated by surgery or radiation therapy. Chemotherapy is used for recurrent or metastatic disease. Radiation is sometimes used together with surgery and/or chemotherapy.

Surgery

Laser surgery and cryosurgery (see Chapter 12) are used to treat precancerous changes and carcinoma in situ, but are not used for invasive cervical cancer. Conization and loop electrosurgical excision procedure (LEEP) (see Chapter 12) can be used to treat precancerous changes and carcinoma in situ.

When the entire cervix must be removed, the surgeon performs an operation called a *hysterectomy*. In a *simple* hysterectomy the

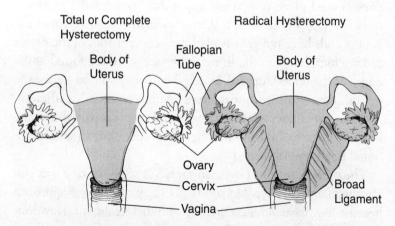

Figure 14.1: Hysterectomy. Shaded areas indicate organs and tissues removed during surgery.

entire uterus (including both the cervix and the body of the uterus) are removed. Surgery to remove both of the ovaries and the fallopian tubes is called a *bilateral salpingo-oophorectomy* (BSO). A BSO is usually done in a postmenopausal woman who needs a hysterectomy. In a radical hysterectomy, the entire uterus, upper vagina, and tissue next to these organs are removed (see Figure 14.1). A *lymphadenectomy*—removal of the nearby lymph nodes—is usually performed with a radical hysterectomy. In any case, a hysterectomy is major surgery that requires general anesthesia and up to a week in the hospital, followed by several weeks of recovery at home.

Most women find they are able to resume their normal activities, including having sexual intercourse, in four to eight weeks. Although menstruation no longer occurs, the ovaries in premenopausal women remain and continue to secrete hormones. Spread of disease to the ovaries is rare, but they are removed in postmenopausal women.

Radiation Therapy

Radiation therapy may be given in one of two ways: (1) from an external source (external beam radiation or teletherapy) similar to the method used to treat breast cancer, or (2) from an internal source (brachytherapy). A capsule containing radioactive material that is inserted into the vagina is the usual form of internal radiation therapy but in some cases, the radioactive material is placed inside thin needles that are placed directly into the tumor.

External radiation treatments are usually given five days a week for four to six weeks. It is not necessary to be hospitalized for the external therapy. Because internal radiation requires special precautions, hospitalization may be necessary for the two or three days in which the implant is in place. However, high dose rate brachytherapy may not require hospitalization because the internal radiation is in place for only a few hours.

When cancer has spread to the regional lymph nodes, radiation therapy is needed to stop multiplication of any cancer cells remaining in the pelvis. Normal cells may be temporarily damaged, but most will eventually recover. For more details on external radiation therapy, see Chapter 8. When any body part is exposed to radiation, similar side effects occur: fatigue and local reactions such as irritation, itching, and burning. However, side effects such as diarrhea, nausea, and vomiting are more common in pelvic radiation. These problems can be treated with medication. Most doctors advise against sexual activity during treatment and for a few weeks afterward, because the tissues may be easily injured and intercourse is likely to be painful. Some women do have lasting side effects, such as vaginal scarring, which can make intercourse difficult. Using vaginal dilators after healing is complete can help prevent vaginal shrinking. Bladder problems include blood in the urine and the need to urinate often. Damage to the ovaries can cause menopausal symptoms in young women. Before undergoing radiation therapy, be sure to discuss all these risks and side effects with your doctor and weigh them against the benefits. You have a choice of radiation therapy or surgery for early-stage cervical cancer. For advanced stages, however, radiation therapy is the only treatment that can cure the cancer. Your doctor and health care team can prevent or treat most of the side effects.

Chemotherapy

Chemotherapy is not a common treatment for cancer of the cervix because most women can be adequately treated with surgery and radiation therapy. However, clinical trials (see Appendix) are under way to evaluate the effectiveness of chemotherapy. Anticancer drugs may be another option when there is a high risk that the cancer will spread; when the cancer has already spread to sites outside the pelvis, such as the lungs; or when the cancer has recurred. Chemotherapy is sometimes used to make cancer cells more vulnerable to radiation therapy or to shrink a large tumor before surgery. Recent clinical trials have found the combination of radiation therapy and chemotherapy more effective than either treatment alone against locally advanced cervical cancers.

The drugs most often used include cisplatin, 5 fluorouracil (5 Fu), bleomycin, and ifosfamide. Some studies have shown that combination therapy with cisplatin and another drug is more toxic than cisplatin alone and is not necessarily more effective for cervical cancer.

CANCER TREATMENT BY STAGE

The following descriptions represent the current standard treatment options in the United States for the stages of cervical cancer.

Carcinoma In Situ

Laser surgery, LEEP, cone biopsy and, less frequently, cryosurgery are all possible treatments for carcinoma in situ. A simple hysterectomy may be considered if the cancer returns, if there is some other uterine condition, or if the woman does not choose to have more children.

An uncommon type of carcinoma in situ called adenocarcinoma in situ is usually treated by hysterectomy. A cone biopsy for adenocarcinoma in situ is considered controversial.

Stage IA

A cone biopsy is an option for removing squamous cell cancers that invade the cervix 3 millimeters (mm) or less (FIGO Stage IA1), especially in women who want to have children. There is a significant risk of recurrence with this type of cancer. Simple hysterectomy is another treatment option for Stage IA1. When cancers have invaded the cervix more deeply than 3 mm (Stage IA2), have spread to lymph nodes or if cancer cells are found inside small lymphatic channels or blood vessels, a radical hysterectomy or radiation therapy is recommended. The ovaries are rarely removed in young women. Over 95 percent of women with Stage IA cervical cancer are cured by these treatments.

Stages IB and IIA

About 90 percent of women with Stage IB and 80 percent of these with Stage IIA cervical cancer are cured by either surgery or radiation therapy—that is, external-beam irradiation (teletherapy) and internal radiation (brachytherapy). Surgery and radiation therapy are equally effective, so the choice will depend greatly on the woman's personal preferences, considering the potential long-term effects of either therapy.

For example, concerns about sexuality are very important, and, compared to radiation therapy, surgery generally interferes less with sexual function. The vagina may be shortened by a hysterectomy, but it remains elastic and capable of lubrication. Radiation therapy, in contrast, does affect the ability of the vagina to expand and become lubricated, though there are treatments to counter these effects.

Surgery also has the advantage of giving the surgeon a view of the pelvic organs and blood vessels, so that lymph nodes around the major blood vessels can be removed *(lymphadenectomy)* and examined to see whether cancer cells are present.

Surgery does have risks. For example, in less than 1 to 2 percent of radical hysterectomies, there is some damage to the urinary tract. And, except for her cancer, a woman has to be in otherwise good health to undergo the operation.

There may be some immediate side effects of radiation therapy—for example, diarrhea, fatigue, and nausea. And some complications take a few years to become apparent. Particularly troublesome are bowel complications such as intestinal obstruction (blockage) or a *fistula*, which is an abnormal connection between the bowel and the vagina, which rarely occur.

Stages IIB, III, and IVA

Radiation therapy (internal and external) is the main treatment option for these advanced stages of cancer of the cervix. Some physicians may also incorporate certain chemotherapy drugs, such as cisplatin, to make the cancer cells more vulnerable to the radiation and recent studies suspect this treatment can prevent or delay cancer recurrence. The combination of chemotherapy and radiation has been shown by recent studies to lengthen the disease-free interval (prevent or delay cancer reoccurence) of women with advanced cervical cancer.

Radiation therapy is the preferred treatment for Stage IVA. In rare situations, a surgeon may recommend an operation that removes all the pelvic reproductive organs *(pelvic exenteration)*, including the vagina, to control the spread of the cancer. Because the surgeon removes the bladder, an *ostomy*, or an opening in the abdominal wall, allows urine to drain from the ureters into an external bag. Another option, a *continent* conduit, is commonly

CERVICAL CANCER IN PREGNANCY

Although cancer of the reproductive organs is rare in pregnant women, when it does occur, cancer of the cervix is more common than any other. In fact, about a third of women diagnosed with this disease are under thirty-five.

Typically, the first step after an abnormal Pap test is colposcopy, just as it is in women who aren't pregnant. The cervix may be larger than normal during pregnancy, but it is still possible to do this visual examination. However, an endocervical curettage (ECC) is not done.

If a precancerous lesion is detected, the health care provider can simply monitor the lesion with colposcopy every few months. The progression from precancer to invasive cancer tends to be slow, and this "watch and wait" approach may be the best option, since progression to cancer is unlikely. If the lesion becomes invasive, studies have shown that a few months' delay poses little risk in terms of survival in women with early cervical cancer. However, consultation with a gynecologic oncologist is advisable.

If the health care provider strongly suspects invasive cancer of the cervix, he or she will consider performing a conization, if the biopsy has failed to show invasive cancer. Pregnancy does increase the possibility of conization complications such as hemorrhage. If done at all, most cone biopsies will be performed in the first or second trimester, but the procedure is rarely done. Nevertheless, a diagnosis of microinvasion on punch biopsy does require a cone biopsy to rule out invasive cancer. The risks to the mother are bleeding and spontaneous abortion. On a more positive note, it's estimated that 80 percent of women who do have this surgery give birth to full-term babies. The cancer does not spread faster, and the fetus is not affected.

Treatment of Stage IB or IIA cancers found during the first half of pregnancy involve termination of the pregnancy. Surgical treatment by hysterectomy will remove the uterus before the fetus can survive outside the womb. The other option, radiation therapy, is lethal to the fetus causing spontaneous abortion. If the pregnancy is beyond twenty weeks, the physician and patient may decide to delay treatment until after cesarean delivery. Stage IIB and more advanced cancers are treated by radiation therapy. If the pregnancy is beyond twenty-four weeks, radiation may be delayed until the fetus can survive outside the womb.

done so that a woman does not have to wear an appliance or ostomy bag. Rather, she learns to periodically drain or catheterize
urine through the stoma, or ostomy opening. When a section of
the colon or rectum is removed, the free ends of the intestine can
be joined to avoid an ostomy for stool.

The five-year survival rates for women with Stage IIB, III, and
IVA cervical cancer are about 65 percent, 40 percent, and 20 percent, respectively.

Stage IVB

Radiation therapy may be helpful in slowing the course of this advanced stage of cervical cancer and giving some pain relief. Clinical trials are under way to test various chemotherapy drugs and
other treatments to slow cancer growth and relieve pain.

Part III
The Uterus

Chapter 15

The Healthy Uterus

The uterus—a hollow, muscular, pear-shaped organ—is suspended deep within the pelvic cavity, between the bladder and the rectum, by an intricate scaffolding of ligaments and muscles. If you imagine the uterus as a pear turned upside down and tilted slightly forward, the rounded end of the pear is called the *fundus*. The middle, widest part is the *corpus* or *body* of the uterus, and the narrow neck is the *cervix*. At this point, the cavity of the uterus merges with the cervical canal, which opens into the vagina (see Chapter 10).

On either side of the uppermost part of the uterus, a *fallopian tube* is positioned above each ovary. Each tube has a funnel-shaped, open end. When an egg is released from one of the ovaries during the menstrual cycle, it passes through the flared, open end of one of the funnels and into that fallopian tube.

The uterus is supplied with blood from the uterine artery and branches of the ovarian artery. Parallel veins carry blood away from the uterus to the hypogastric and uterine veins.

The uterus or womb holds and nourishes the developing fetus, and its powerful muscular layer contracts during labor to force the baby out of the uterus through the birth canal. The three layers that form the strong uterine wall are the thin outer *serous* coat or *serosa*; the thick middle layer, called the *myometrium* or muscular coat; and the innermost layer, the *endometrium* (Figure 15.1). Lymph vessels drain lymphatic fluid from the myometrium to the network of channels along the supporting ligaments and the fallopian tubes. In this chapter, we will be focusing primarily on the endometrium, which is where 97 percent of uterine body and fundus cancers develop.

The inner layer of the uterus is made up of endometrial epithelial cells. The endometrium also consists of connective tissue called *stroma*. The superficial endometrial layer is sometimes called the *functional* layer, because it goes through predictable changes each month in response to hormonal stimulation from estrogen and progesterone. The deeper part of the endometrium is called the basal layer.

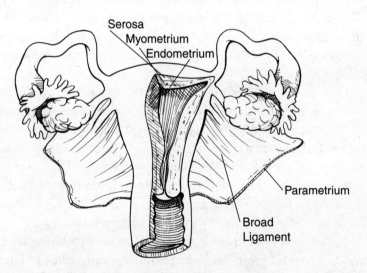

Serosa
Myometrium
Endometrium
Parametrium
Broad
Ligament

Figure 15.1: Cross-section of the uterus.

The menstrual cycle begins when epithelial cells in the deepest layer of the endometrium proliferate and push up to the functional layer. At the same time, blood vessels called spiral arterioles are developing to supply the new cells with nutrients. These changes are orchestrated by the hormones to prepare the uterus to receive and nourish a fertilized egg. If that fails to happen, *menstruation* occurs—that is, the new blood vessels constrict and degenerate, curtailing the blood supply to the endometrium, so the new cells die and are sloughed off, and the glands that are interspersed throughout the lining collapse. The mix of dead tissue and blood, called *menses*, exits through the cervical canal into the vagina.

It's important to understand the impact of hormonal stimulation on the endometrium, because the activity of estrogen and progesterone is believed to partially influence the development of cancer. Estrogen causes the cells of the endometrium to multiply and, to a lesser extent, stimulates the production of cells in the myometrium. Simultaneously, estrogen stimulates the production of progesterone receptors on the cells, so that they become more sensitive to that hormone. Progesterone causes maturation of the cells. The net effect of this stimulation is that the endometrial cells become larger, and the glands interspersed throughout this layer increase their secretion.

WHAT IS UTERINE CANCER?

Cancer in the epithelial lining of the uterus—also called endometrial cancer or *endometrial adenocarcinoma*—is the most common gynecologic cancer and the fourth most common cancer in women.

How or why cancer begins in the uterus is not exactly known, but several risk factors have been identified, and researchers are making progress in understanding how these factors cause endometrial tissue to become cancerous. The incidence of endometrial cancer is greatest in women who have gone through menopause or who, for any of a variety of reasons, have an excess of estrogen relative to progesterone. This imbalance causes endometrial cells to grow too much. An adequate amount of progesterone would allow the glands to mature and stop cell overgrowth.

Obese women, women with fertility problems, and women who do not ovulate at each menstrual cycle tend to have a hormonal imbalance (too much estrogen relative to the amount of progesterone) that increases their risk of developing endometrial cancer. Women who are fifty or more pounds overweight, for example, have ten times the risk for endometrial cancer, compared to women of normal weight. Interestingly, the adrenal glands, which sit on top of the kidneys, produce a hormone called androstenedione that is converted to a weak estrogen (estrone) by fat cells. So even though a women is in menopause, she can still produce estrogen but not progesterone. Similarly, if she takes estrogen replacement therapy without supplemental progesterone, the uterine glands will be overstimulated. In fact, following the 1960s and 1970s, when estrogen replacement therapy was given without progesterone, there was an increased incidence of uterine lining, or endometrial, cancer. According to a study conducted during the late 1970s and early 1980s, the risk of endometrial cancer among long-term users of estrogen alone was four times to eight times greater.

Scientists suspect that several other risk factors, such as eating a high-fat diet, having a pattern of abnormal menstruation (especially increased bleeding at the time of menopause), late menopause (after age fifty-two), diabetes, and high blood pressure, may also alter the balance of estrogen and progresterone, causing increased growth of endometrial cells.

There is an association between the drug tamoxifen, which is used to treat or prevent breast cancer, and an increased risk of endometrial cancer. Although tamoxifen blocks estrogen's affects on breast tissue, the drug mimics the effect of estrogen in stimulating endometrial cell growth. However, because the benefits of the anticancer therapy outweigh the risks of developing cancer in the uterus, tamoxifen therapy is usually given to women with breast cancer, and less often, to women of high risk of developing breast cancer. But they are monitored closely to detect endometrial cancer early (see Chapter 16). The progression of endometrial hyperplasia to cancer does not account for all of the cases of endometrial cancer, so experts argue that there must be some other explanation for a uterine malignancy. It is known also that endometrial cancer can occur in a uterus that appears normal and has no hyperplasia.

Not all endometrial cancer risk factors are related to hormone balance, however. Women with a strong family history of endometrial cancer are at increased risk. In some cancer, this familial risk is believed to be due to inherited mutations in genes responsible for DNA repair. Inherited defects in these genes are also associated with an increased risk of colorectal cancer. Women with a family history that raises the possibility of the inherited syndrome, called hereditary nonpolyposis colon cancer (HNPCC) should ask their physicians about genetic counseling and the possible benefits and disadvantages of genetic testing.

Most estrogen-related endometrial cancers develop over a period of years. Many are known to follow and possibly develop from less serious abnormalities of the endometrium.

Endometrial hyperplasia is an increased growth of the endometrium that, like endometrial cancer, is often due to a hormonal imbalance. Endometrial hyperplasia is classified as *simple* or *complex* based on the shape of endometrial glands, and as *without atypia* or *with atypia* based on features of the individual cells that form these glands. Combining these features together yields the four types of hyperplasia, which are important to distinguish from one another. Women with some types have a substantial risk of later developing endometrial cancer, whereas the risk is quite low for other types. These risks for *simple hyperplasia without atypia, complex hyperplasia without atypia, simple hyperplasia with atypia* and *complex hyperplasia with atypia* are 1 percent, 3 percent, 8 percent, and 29 percent, respectively. Fortunately, endometrial hyperplasia can usually be effectively treated to prevent cancer from developing. A hysterectomy is usually recommended for postmenopausal women who have complex hyperplasia with atypia.

PREVENTING ENDOMETRIAL CANCER

Premenopausal women who have an abnormal buildup of endometrial tissue (hyperplasia) may be placed on hormone (progestin) therapy for about two weeks of each menstrual cycle, for several months. If irregular periods persist, oral contraceptives containing both estrogen and progestin may be prescribed to create a normal cycle. Oral contraceptives decrease the risk of endometrial cancer. A physician may recommend hysterectomy for a woman who has hyperplasia with atypia who has completed her family or has entered menopause.

The most important preventive step for menopausal women who are taking estrogen replacement therapy is to also take progesterone. The exception is a woman has had her uterus removed by a hysterectomy.

SCREENING TESTS

There is currently no recommended test for detecting endometrial cancer in healthy women with no symptoms. The Pap test is an excellent screening test for cervical cancer but is much less accurate in detecting endometrial cancer. It will often detect endometrial cancer that has spread to the cervix but will miss most early endometrial cancers. Palpating the uterus during the pelvic exam is not likely to detect a tumor either, because a malignancy does not usually alter the size or shape of the organ in the early stages of the disease. Retrieving samples of the endometrium for microscopic examination—an *endometrial biopsy*—is often recommended for women who are experiencing symptoms such as spotting, heavy menstrual bleeding, or bleeding after menopause. It is sometimes recommended for women with certain risk factors, but it is not recommended as a routine screening test.

Chapter 16

Diagnosis and Staging

A malignancy in the uterus usually signals its presence with a noticeable symptom: vaginal discharge. Eighty percent of the time, abnormal bleeding occurs. Occasionally, a woman will experience a sensation of pressure in her pelvis. When the disease is advanced, a woman may also lose weight, feel weak, and tire easily.

When bleeding occurs as a result of uterine cancer, it is usually because the lining of the uterus, the endometrium, has been disrupted by a tumor. Unfortunately, some women delay detection of the cancer by ignoring the irregular bleeding. When the discharge is brought to a gynecologist's attention, uterine cancer is one of the first conditions suspected, especially in a woman who has gone through menopause. It's estimated that one-third of the cases of vaginal bleeding in older women are due to cancer; in younger women, bleeding is far less likely to be caused by cancer and is usually the result of some hormonal imbalance.

DIAGNOSTIC TESTS

Endometrial Biopsy

To investigate the cause of the bleeding, the physician will remove a small amount of tissue in a procedure called *endometrial* or *aspiration biopsy*.

Tissue samples from the uterus can be obtained through a suction catheter inserted through the cervix into the uterus. This is an office procedure. Although it is uncomfortable for a brief moment, the pain may be relieved some by taking a nonnarcotic analgesic such as a nonsteroidal antiinflammatory agent (ibuprofen, for example). Afterward, there will be some bleeding for a day or two. If the tissue contains cancer cells, no further diagnostic tests are needed.

Dilation and Curettage

If the results of endometrial biopsy are not conclusive and the physician feels a larger tissue sample is necessary, he or she may perform *dilation and curettage* (D & C) with or without hysteroscopy. A general anesthetic or a local anesthetic plus intravenous sedation is used. The gynecologist dilates the cervix and scapes the inside of the cervix (endocervix) and the lining of the uterus (endometrium), with a small curette, a spoon-shaped instrument that has a cutting edge. The tissue obtained in this way can be examined under a microscope for detection of any cancer cells.

A hospital stay following the procedure is not necessary. There may be some bleeding and mild cramping for a few days.

Other Tests

Using a technique known as *hysteroscopy*, the gynecologist inserts a viewing instrument into the uterus and visually examines the lining. Or, a transvaginal sonogram (see Chapter 18) may indicate whether a tumor is present and whether it extends into the myometrium.

Another diagnostic test is an *ultrahysterosonogram* or *saline infusion sonogram*. Saline is introduced into the uterus through a catheter before the transvaginal sonogram is done. This will allow the doctor to see abnormalities of the uterine lining.

If the pathologist examining the endometrial biopsy or D & C specimen determines that cancer is present, the next step is surgery to remove the uterus. First, though, some tests are necessary to determine whether the cancer has spread to other organs. These tests typically include a chest X-ray and some routine blood tests. If the blood tests suggest that liver metastasis may be present, a CT scan will be done to check for masses inside the liver.

CA-125 is a substance released into the bloodstream by many endometrial and ovarian cancers. Very high blood CA-125 levels suggest that an endometrial cancer has probably spread beyond the uterus. CA-125 measurements are also useful because, if levels are elevated, followup measurements can be used to estimate the effectiveness of treatment (levels will drop if treatment is effective) and to identify cancer recurrence after initially successful treatment. However, this test is not routinely performed.

Studies are in progress to determine whether ultrasonography or MRI scans are useful in predicting whether endometrial cancer has invaded the muscle layer of the uterine wall (myometrium) or if it has spread to lymph nodes, but these tests are not used routinely.

If a woman has symptoms or signs suggesting spread of endometrial cancer to the bladder or rectum, the inside of these organs can be viewed through a lighted tube, in examinations called cystoscopy and proctoscopy. If spread around the ureters (the tubes that connect the kidneys to the bladder) is suspected, an *intravenous pyelogram* or *IVP* may be done. This is an X-ray test that outlines the urinary system. A computed tomography (CT) scan with contrast will provide the same information and is used more often than an IVP.

TYPES OF UTERINE CANCER

This section of the book is devoted to the most common type of cancer of the body of the uterus—adenocarcinoma of the endometrium. There are other types, and some are more aggressive than others. For all types, however, hysterectomy is the usual treatment. The types of uterine cancer include:

- Epithelial cancer (endometrioid adenocarcinoma, adenosquamous carcinoma, clear cell carcinoma, papillary serous carcinoma), which forms in the lining layer, or *epithelium*, of the uterus.
- Uterine sarcomas, which include stromal sarcomas and malignant mixed mesodermal tumors or carcinosarcomas (which develop in the connective tissue of the endometrium), and leiomyosarcomas (which start in the muscular wall of the uterus).

SURGICAL STAGING

If endometrial cancer is present, the uterus must be removed in a hysterectomy. As described in Section II, this operation includes removal of the body of the uterus as well as the cervix. The ovaries and fallopian tubes are usually removed as well. During the operation, the surgeon will obtain samples of fluid from the pelvis and abdomen, and from under the *diaphragm* (the muscle that separates the chest from the abdomen). Small biopsies may rarely be taken of the *peritoneum* (a layer of tissue that lines the abdomen and pelvis). These samples are checked microscopically for cancer cells.

The surgeon may make the incision for the hysterectomy through the abdomen or it may be possible to remove the reproductive organs through an incision in the vagina. The latter is called a *vaginal hysterectomy*. Survival rates for each approach are similar. Some surgeons use a periscope-like instrument called a *laparoscope*, which allows them to view the pelvic cavity and remove lymph nodes, along with the reproductive organs, through a vaginal incision.

The uterus is sent to the hospital pathology laboratory and a pathologist will determine the tumor grade and whether the cancer has invaded the muscle of the uterine wall (and, if so, how deeply) or has spread to the cervix. This evaluation takes about 15 minutes and is done while the patient is still under anesthesia in the operating room. If the cancer has spread to the cervix, has invaded more than halfway through the uterine wall, or is Grade 2 or 3, the surgeon will then remove some lymph nodes from the pelvis, and others near the large blood vessels (paraaortic lymph nodes), for examination. Regardless of the cancer's grade and depth of invasion, any large lymph nodes noted during the operation will be removed. If the cancer is a uterine papillary serous cell carcinoma, the large fold of fatty tissue that covers the pelvic organs, the *omentum*, may be removed also.

Because of the need to perform these specialized procedures, a gynecologic oncologist should be present or available for the surgery. The surgery may be modified if the woman is generally not in good health, in addition to having the cancer. Very obese women or those with heart disease or other serious health problems may not be able to tolerate such extensive surgery.

STAGING

After the surgery is done and the laboratory reports are complete, the surgeon can establish the extent of the cancer. As with the

Staging for Endometrial Cancer

FIGO Stage   *Description*

I Cancer limited to corpus (body of the uterus).
   IA Cancer limited to endometrium (lining layer of the corpus).
   IB Invasion of less than half of the myometrium (muscle layer of the uterus).
   IC Invasion of more than half of the myometrium.
  Each case is also graded as G1, G2, or G3. Grading will be based on nuclear/cytoplasmic feature (such as the size and shape of the cells), as well as the extent of arrangement of these cells into glands.

II Involvement of the cervix and the corpus.
   IIA Endocervical glandular involvement only.
   IIB Cervical stromal (connective tissue) involvement.
  Each case will be graded as G1, G2, or G3.

III Spread outside of the uterus, confined to pelvis (not including bladder or rectal involvement).
   IIIA Involvement of uterine serosa (the thin layer that covers the outer surface of the uterus); *adnexa* (the ovaries, fallopian tubes, and/or the ligaments that hold the uterus); and/or cancer cells are found in the pelvic cavity.
   IIIB Spread to the vagina.
   IIIC Spread to *retroperitoneal lymph nodes.*
  Each case will be graded as G1, G2, or G3.

IV Spread to the bladder, rectum, distant sites.
   IVA Involvement of bladder and/or rectal mucosa.
   VB Spread beyond the pelvic organs to *inguinal* (groin area) lymph nodes, to organs of the abdomen, and to other distant organs.
  Each case will be graded as G1, G2, or G3.

other gynecologic cancers, the stage will determine what subsequent treatment, if any, is needed.

In 1988, the International Federation of Obstetrics and Gynecology (FIGO) updated its staging system to incorporate the pathology of the tumor (its appearance under the microscope) as well as the anatomic extent of the disease (how far the cancer has spread). Tumors are defined as Grade (G) 1, 2, or 3, depending on how close to normal the tumor cells are, and how well the tumor cells form glands that resemble normal endometrial glands. G1 is *well differentiated* (there is a close similarity to normal cells and glands); G2 is *moderately differentiated*; and G3 is *poorly differentiated* (the cells are quite abnormal and there is very little gland formation). The box on page 195 describes the four stages of endometrial cancer.

Chapter 17

Treatment of Endometrial Cancer

Endometrial cancer is one of the most curable cancers if it is di-agnosed early. The overall five-year survival rate for all stages combined is about 84 percent.

SURGERY

Surgery to remove the body of the uterus and the cervix (a *total hysterectomy*), along with removal of both of the fallopian tubes and ovaries (bilateral salpingo-oophorectomy), is almost always the first step in confirming the diagnosis, staging the disease, and treat-ing it (see Chapter 16). In many cases, nearby lymph nodes and a sample of omentum are also removed. Surgery is the primary treat-ment for more than 90 percent of women with endometrial can-cer. From that point on, however, treatment plans vary, based on the extent of the cancer and how fast-growing it appears to be.

RADIATION THERAPY

Radiation therapy (RT) before surgery, to shrink a large tumor, was once a standard treatment, but now preoperative RT is not usually done. If the cancer has been detected early, radiation therapy may not be necessary, and some experts feel that prescrib-ing it before surgery is overtreating the disease.

For a small group of women—less than 5 to 10 percent—who have advanced cancer or are not in good health, radiation therapy *instead* of surgery may be the treatment of choice. This approach is especially useful in elderly women who have other serious medical problems that make surgery very risky. However, consultation with a gynecologic oncologist is essential before treatment with RT alone.

Brachytherapy

How much of the pelvis needs to be exposed to radiation therapy depends on the extent of the disease. In cases where only the upper third of the vagina—the *vaginal cuff*—needs to be treated, a radioactive implant is employed. This internal application of radiation therapy is called *brachytherapy.*

Four to six weeks after the hysterectomy, the surgeon or radiation oncologist inserts a special applicator into the woman's vagina in the radiation suite of the hospital or care center, and pellets of radioactive material are inserted into the applicator. Several treatments may be necessary. With vaginal brachytherapy, there is little radiation effect on nearby structures, such as the bladder or rectum.

If cancer cells are present in the fluid sampled during surgery, then a radioactive solution, such as radioactive phosphate, may be introduced through a catheter into the abdominal and pelvic cavities after the surgery. Treatment with this radioactive solution should not be combined with external beam radiation therapy.

External Beam Radiation Therapy

If the cancer has extended more than half way through the myometrium or is a Grade 3 cancer, indicating a potential for lymph node involvement, or if microscopic examination of lymph nodes found cancer cells, the entire pelvis is usually treated with external beam radiation therapy. Depending on the location of affected lymph nodes, the radiation field may be extended to also include the abdomen (paraaortic field). This is the more familiar type of therapy in which the radiation is delivered from an outside source. In some situations, both brachytherapy and external beam RT are given sequentially.

This more common type of RT requires four to five weeks of five-days-a-week treatment. As in breast cancer (see Chapter 8), the area to be exposed to radiation is carefully marked with permanent ink or injected dye similar to a tattoo. A special mold of the pelvis and lower back is custom-made to ensure that the woman is placed in the exact same position for each treatment.

The actual treatment takes less than a half hour, but the daily visits to the radiation center may be tiring and inconvenient. Serious fatigue, which may not occur until two weeks after therapy begins, is a common side effect. As the radiation passes through the skin to its intended target, it may damage the skin cells. This is rare; but when it happens, the irritation ranges from temporary and mild redness to permanent discoloration. The skin may release fluid, which can lead to infection, so care must be taken to clean and protect the area exposed to radiation. (See Chapter 8 for specific information on what can and cannot be used on skin, and other special precautions.) Diarrhea is a common side effect, but it can usually be controlled with nonprescription medications such as Immodium or Lomotil. Irritation to the bladder (radiation cystitis) may also occur, resulting in discomfort and an urge to urinate frequently.

CHEMOTHERAPY

Chemotherapy is designed to kill cancer cells throughout the body. With uterine cancer, chemotherapy drugs can shrink a tumor, at least temporarily, in 35 to 40 percent of women. Studies have not yet shown that this treatment helps women to survive longer.

In general, combinations of drugs appear more effective than a single drug in temporarily shrinking the cancer, but they do not seem to improve overall survival. Drugs typically used for women with advanced cancer are doxorubicin, cyclophosphamide, cisplatin, and carboplatin. Paclitaxel is also being used. (See Chapter 20 for more information about these drugs.) New drugs, as well as new combinations of current drugs, are being tested in clinical trials and are a good option for some women with advanced or recurrent endometrial cancer.

Hormone therapy with progestins appears to be as effective as some of the chemotherapy drugs in women whose cancers are well differentiated (Grade 1) and have progesterone and estrogen receptors. Tests to determine whether these receptors are present can be done on the same sample of the cancer removed by a biopsy or by the hysterectomy. Hormone therapy may be recommended when cancer recurs, particularly if hormone receptors are present.

Tamoxifen, a drug that blocks the action of estrogen, has yielded a 15 to 20 percent response rate in women with metastatic or recurrent endometrial cancer.

TREATMENT BY STAGE OF ENDOMETRIAL CANCER

Stage I

A simple hysterectomy plus the removal of both ovaries and fallopian tubes (bilateral salpingo-oophorectomy, or BSO) are done, and, depending on the extent and grade of the cancer, selected lymph nodes are removed and examined for cancer. If the cancer is Grade 1 and either does not invade the myometrium or has penetrated less than one third to halfway through that layer, routine lymph node sampling is not done. Any abnormally large nodes will still be removed, however. Samples of tissue from the omentum may also be examined for cancer cells.

If the cancer is Grade 1 and no lymph nodes are involved, radiation therapy may not be done. However, if the cancer is Grade 2 or 3, or if the cancer extends through more than half of the wall of the uterus, radiation therapy may be given to the area to lower the risk of local recurrence.

Progestin therapy may be especially useful in young women with early-stage uterine cancer who want to have children. This experimental treatment may cause the cancer to regress, allowing a full-term pregnancy to occur, but this approach is very controversial and it is not without risks. A second opinion from a gynecologic oncologist and pathologist (to be certain about the cancer's grade) before progestin therapy is important.

The average 5-year survival rate for women with Stage I endometrial cancer is 75 percent. The rate is somewhat higher for those with Grade 1 cancers and lower if the cancer is Grade 3.

Stage II

If spread to the cervix is detectable only by examining tissue under the microscope the standard treatment is a simple hysterectomy and BSO (see above). If the cancer visibly (grossly) extends to the cervix, a radical hysterectomy and BSO, or a simple hysterectomy and preoperative radiation is necessary. In either case, the pelvic and paraaortic lymph nodes are usually sampled and examined for cancer cells.

Radiation therapy—internal and external—may also be given after surgery. The average 5-year survival rate is 60 to 70 percent.

Stage III

If all visible cancer can be removed, a hysterectomy and BSO are performed, and pelvic and paraaortic lymph nodes may be removed. The surgery is followed with radiation therapy.

If it is not possible to remove all the cancer, surgery may not be performed, and radiation therapy is the standard treatment. Sometimes, radiation will shrink the cancer enough that attempts to completely remove it are worthwhile. Women with Stage III cancer are encouraged to enter a clinical trial evaluating chemotherapy, hormonal therapy or other new treatments. The 5-year survival rate is about 50 percent.

Stage IV

A hysterectomy and BSO are sometimes done, not to cure the disease but to prevent excessive bleeding or other local complications. Radiation therapy may be done for the same reason. Hormone therapy is also an option. Women with Stage IV cancer are encouraged to enter a clinical trial evaluating chemotherapy or other new treatments. Depending on the extent of spread within the abdomen and to distant organs, the 5-year survival rate will vary from 10 to 30 percent.

Recurrent Cancer

Treatment depends on the amount and location of the cancer. Usual options include radiation, hormonal therapy, chemotherapy, and clinical trials of new treatments.

Part IV

The Ovaries

Chapter 18

The Healthy Ovary

Each of the two ovaries is about the size and shape of an almond. An ovary is suspended on each side of the uterus, where it is held in place by several ligaments. Arteries, veins, lymph vessels, and nerves criss-cross these ligaments to reach the ovaries.

The two ovaries are the female hormone factories of a woman's body. The estrogen and progesterone the ovaries produce are in part responsible for maintaining many of the physical characteristics that we associate with femininity. These hormones control the development of the breasts, and they help regulate the menstrual cycle.

Each ovary contains thousands of *follicles,* each of which contains an *oocyte* or egg. During the childbearing years, a *gonadotropin-releasing hormone* in the brain stimulates the pituitary gland at the base of the brain to release *follicle-stimulating hormone,* which in turn stimulates the growth of a few follicles in the ovary (Figure 18.1). One of them will respond by growing and filling with fluid, eventually forming a cystic swelling on the ovary. Within the follicle, the oocyte is also growing larger, and the cells lining the follicle produce estrogen. During *ovulation,* the follicle and its egg finally bursts through the layer of cells covering the ovary, called the *germinal epithelium.*

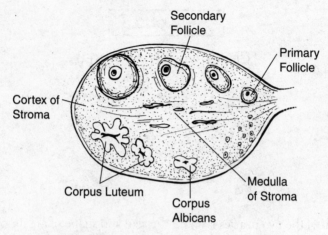

Figure 18.1: Cross-section of an ovary.

The follicle collapses and the tear in the ovary's surface begins to heal. But the follicle's work is not done when it ruptures and releases the egg. The collapsed follicle, now called the *corpus luteum,* begins to produce progesterone and some estrogen. If the egg is not fertilized by a sperm cell, the corpus luteum starts to turn into scar tissue at the end of that monthly cycle. This cycle is repeated every 28 days or so. If the egg is fertilized and pregnancy ensues, the corpus luteum remains for several months and it will supply the hormones needed to maintain the pregnancy.

WHO IS AT RISK FOR OVARIAN CANCER?

Cancer is the excessive proliferation and spread of abnormal cells. Because the ovary is an organ characterized by monthly cycles of intense cell production, some experts believe that the number of times a woman ovulates is linked to her cancer risk. Every month, after the egg is released, the epithelial cells must multiply to heal the wound created by the ruptured follicle. The more often this happens, one theory goes, the greater the possibility of error in the cells' molecular machinery, and the greater the risk of altered cells. This may turn out to be a very simplistic model, however, especially in view of new knowledge gained from molecular biology.

Fertility

Having children seems to reduce one's risk of ovarian cancers. According to one study, the birth of each child reduces a woman's risk of ovarian cancer by 14 percent. Other research has shown that it's actually the number of pregnancies that's important, even if those pregnancies result in miscarriage. Taking birth control pills, which hormonally resembles pregnancy and suppresses ovulation, also considerably lowers a woman's risk of ovarian cancer.

These observations led researchers to consider that excessive ovulation or high levels of gonadotropins, were causes of ovarian cancer. Interestingly, a conflicting study, done in 1993, revealed that tubal sterilization (cutting or "tying" the tubes) offered some protection against ovarian cancer. Ovulation still occurred, but pregnancy was prevented. However, the protective effect of tubal sterilization may involve a different mechanism—blocking passage of cancer-causing chemicals from the vagina or uterus that would otherwise reach the ovaries through the tubes. This theory remains unproven.

Hormone Therapies

Several studies indicate that infertility treatments that involve ovulation-stimulating hormonal therapies are linked to ovarian

205705

208281

cancer, and there have been reports of young women developing ovarian cancer during or after infertility treatment. However, critics of these studies say there are several shortcomings in this research. For instance, it's not clear why the women were infertile. Perhaps some underlying condition was linked to the ovarian cancer. Also, some of the studies were too small to be considered statistically valid, so the link is still quite questionable.

Some studies have suggested long-term use of postmenopausal estrogen replacement therapy (ERT) may be associated with increased risk of ovarian cancer. According to a study of 240,000 women, the longer a woman took the hormone, the more her risk increased. However, the researchers pointed out that this study was done at a time when women took much larger doses of estrogen than are now typically prescribed. Furthermore, today, women often take progesterone in addition to estrogen, which may counteract some of the latter's effects. This and other risks of ERT, as well as the benefits of ERT are not the same in all women. Decisions regarding ERT should take a woman's medical individual situation into account.

Genetics

Family history plays a role in only about 7 percent of women with ovarian cancer. The risk of developing ovarian cancer increases from 1.8 percent in a woman who has no family history to 7 percent in those who have two relatives with the disease. Since the discovery of the BRCA 1 gene (a breast cancer susceptibility gene that is also linked to ovarian cancer), researchers have determined that about 1 in 200 American women carry a mutated form of the gene (see Chapter 4). Inheriting a BRCA 1 mutation increases a woman's lifetime risk of developing ovarian cancer by up to 40 percent. Women with BRCA 1 mutations are predisposed to ovarian cancer in their mid-forties and mid-fifties whereas sporadic (not inherited) cases usually are found in women over sixty. The BRCA 2 gene, another breast cancer susceptibility gene, has also been linked to ovarian cancer, and it has been reported (though not confirmed) that a woman with the BRCA 2 gene has about a 15 percent chance of developing ovarian cancer.

A far less common inherited disorder is Lynch Syndrome II or hereditary nonpolyposis colorectal cancer (HNPCC), a form of colorectal cancer that increases one's risk of developing cancer in other organs, such as the ovaries and uterus (see Chapter 15).

The number and age of female relatives affected by ovarian or breast cancer is the main criterion for determining whether a woman is at risk for developing hereditary ovarian cancer. Women who have three first-degree relatives with ovarian cancer are considered to be at high risk for the disease, and some doctors suggest having these women's ovaries removed surgically (oophorectomy) as soon as their family is complete. Others suggest testing for mutations of the BRCA 1 and BRCA 2 genes before proceeding with an oophorectomy. However, research has shown that this surgery does not guarantee freedom from cancer. There is a rare type of cancer known as *peritoneal papillary serous carcinoma* or *extraovarian serous carcinoma* that, in many respects, is similar to ovarian cancer. But this cancer can develop from tissue remaining in the pelvis even after both ovaries have been removed. Nevertheless, it's estimated that *prophylactic oophorectomy*—preventive removal of the ovaries—would result in a 50 percent reduction in ovarian cancers.

Women who have a family member with any type of hereditary breast or ovarian cancer can benefit from talking about their family history with a genetic counseler. Some women may request genetic tests to determine whether they carry the BRCA 1 or BRCA 2 gene. Even if they don't have the genetic tests, their best protection is to have careful cancer screening, perhaps done more often or begun at a younger age than women without such a family history. Some experts recommend transvaginal ultrasound and tumor markers, starting at about age twenty-five to thirty. However, as noted earlier, the effectiveness of these tests for early detection is uncertain.

Habits

It has long been suspected that talcum powder applied to the genital area or used on products that come into contact with the genitals, such as a diaphragm and sanitary napkins, is linked to ovarian cancer. Recently, a study of more than 700 women showed that those who used genital sprays had a 90 percent increased risk of developing ovarian cancer. Not all of the sprays contained talc (a silicate of magnesium), so the researchers speculate that perhaps some other ingredient is responsible. In this study, women who used body powder—cornstarch, talcum powder, baby powder, deodorant powder, and bath powder—in the genital area had a 60 percent increased risk, but using one of these products on a diaphragm or on sanitary napkins did not have a similar effect. This study is far from conclusive, though, because the scientists depended on the women's memory of their habits, which is not the most accurate source. Although the evidence is far from conclusive, it seems reasonable to avoid these products.

In 1995, the results of the first large study of diet and ovarian cancer were published. The disease was linked to high levels of saturated fat in the diet. According to an analysis involving about 1,000 women, the risk of ovarian cancer increased 20 percent for every 10 grams of saturated fat consumed daily. (A tablespoon of butter is 8 grams; a three-ounce hamburger is 7 grams.) The study also revealed that the risk could be lowered by eating vegetables: a half-cup of vegetables decreased the risk by the same amount. Other studies have not confirmed these data, but eating a low fat diet with five to six servings of fruits and vegetables a day is the foundation for a healthy diet that is known to reduce the risk of several other diseases.

It is not known why saturated fat might have such an impact on ovarian cancer risk or why eating vegetables might lower it, but researchers speculate that estrogen is involved in some way. Saturated fat may contain estrogen or may increase a woman's estrogen production. Some plants contain "phytoestrogens." When they are consumed, the ovaries may get a signal to slow down their estrogen production. Fiber in vegetables may also play some role.

SCREENING TESTS

Screening tests simply are not yet accurate enough to warrant their widespread use, so they are indicated only for women at high risk of developing ovarian cancer. Therefore, when experts discuss attempts at screening for this cancer, they usually refer mainly to women with two or more first-degree relatives with ovarian cancer and women with known BRCA gene mutations. Tests for ovarian cancer should also be done for women who have symptoms such as lower abdominal pain, swelling, or bloating, which might be a warning sign of this disease.

Ultrasonography

Ultrasound is the use of high-frequency sound waves to create an image of internal organs. For *vaginal ultrasound*, also called *transvaginal sonography* (TVS), the sound waves are delivered through a wandlike instrument inserted into the vagina (Figure 18.2). As sound waves bounce off the nearby ovaries, uterus, and fallopian tubes, a computer converts the echo into an image that can be studied. This relatively painless test can be done in a few minutes in a doctor's office, and it is less expensive than other imaging tests such as computed tomography (CT scanning) and magnetic resonance imaging (MRI).

Transvaginal sonography can detect an abnormal mass on an ovary, indicating the possibility of a tumor, but it does not reveal whether the mass is a benign cyst or a cancer. Still, TVS is a more accurate test than a pelvic examination, in which the physician attempts to feel an abnormal lesion on an ovary.

Recently, some advances in imaging technology have produced some useful tests. For example, a technique that measures blood flow in vessels that supply the ovaries, called *color flow Doppler imaging*, displays a pattern of the circulation. When used

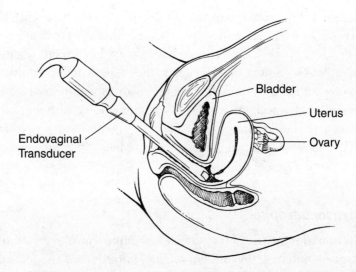

Figure 18.2: Procedure for vaginal ultrasound study.

in conjunction with TVS, it can indicate whether abnormal vessels have formed, a common feature of a malignant tumor. (However, increased blood flow also occurs with benign ovarian cysts.)

Tumor Markers

Scientists have learned how to identify and accurately measure certain proteins produced by cancer cells that circulate in the bloodstream. One of these *tumor markers*, CA-125, is present in about 80 percent of women with ovarian cancer, which makes it a useful indicator of a therapy's effectiveness and of ovarian cancer's recurrence after treatment.

In the late 1980s, scientists learned that CA-125 is sometimes elevated just before some ovarian cancers begin to cause symptoms, so it was hoped that a blood test for the marker could detect the disease in women who had no other signs or symptoms. Unfortunately, the test wasn't sensitive enough. Less than half the women with early-stage ovarian cancer had an elevated CA-125 level. CA-125 can rise during menstruation and pregnancy and when other common conditions, such as endometriosis or fibroids, are present. Considering the high proportion of women who would be subjected to exploratory surgery unnecessarily, a test for CA-125 is not recommended for routine screening.

Blood levels of other tumor markers, such as CA-19-9 and carcinoembryonric antigen (CEA) are sometimes elevated in patients with the mucinous type of epithelial ovarian cancers. Human chorionic gonadotropin (HCG) and/or alpha fetoprotein (AFP) levels are increased in some germ cell ovarian cancers. As in the case of CA-125, these markers are sometimes useful in assessing a woman's response to treatment or early detection of recurrence after treatment, but they are not recommended as routine screening tests.

In 1994, a National Institute of Health consensus panel concluded that no currently available test—not CA-125 or ultrasound—detected a sufficient number of ovarian cancers among a low-risk group of women to warrant use as a screening test.

The search for another tumor marker continues, and many studies of other products of ovarian cancer cells are under way.

Chapter 19

Is It Ovarian Cancer?

Perhaps more than for any other gynecologic malignancy, early diagnosis of ovarian cancer is critical for survival. The five-year survival rate for women diagnosed with early-stage disease is about 90 percent. Unfortunately, more than 75 percent of women with ovarian cancer are diagnosed when regional or distant spread of the disease is already present. Five-year survival for women whose cancer has spread beyond an ovary to the lymph nodes and distant sites is about 25 percent.

One reason why early diagnosis is so difficult is that the ovaries are deep in the pelvic cavity and are well protected (and hidden) by the layers of tissue surrounding them. Signs and symptoms that indicate one of the ovaries is diseased may not become obvious until the tumor is large. When symptoms do occur, they tend to be vague and nonspecific, and a woman may tolerate them for some time before seeing a doctor. Physicians also may not recognize that the symptoms are caused by an ovarian cancer rather than some benign condition.

Symptoms may include pelvic pain or generalized abdominal discomfort, low back pain, persistent bloating, frequent urination, and digestive problems, such as loss of appetite, a feeling of fullness, gas, and constipation. Severe vomiting and significant weight loss are also signs of advanced disease.

DETECTING THE TUMOR

When an abnormality is suspected, the initial tests to confirm a tumor or cyst may include transvaginal ultrasound and color flow Doppler imaging. CA-125 is especially useful in evaluating a postmenopausal woman with symptoms or a pelvic mass.

If the physician is fairly certain there is a tumor, a closer look at the mass may be achieved with ultrasonography. Computed tomography (CT or CAT scan) or magnetic resonance imaging (MRI) can also evaluate the mass, but these tests are better at detecting abnormalities in surrounding structures. Both tests provide images of soft tissue, so the ovaries and other organs of the pelvis can be visualized. A CT scan involves some radiation exposure because it relies on X-rays of the body. A computer converts these views into a cross-sectional image. An MRI does not use X-rays but relies on radio waves to make its detailed cross-sectional pictures. An imaging test can only detect an abnormal growth. To find out whether the growth is cancerous, a biopsy must be done to retrieve a sample of tissue from the tumor for analysis under a microscope. If cancer is found, these same tests can be used again later, to gauge the effectiveness of treatment or to detect any recurrence of the cancer.

A newer but very expensive technique is positron-emission tomography (PET scan), which involves injecting a very small amount of a radioactive substance into the bloodstream and using an apparatus to record the radioactive emissins from the organ being scanned. A computer translates the data into an image. The PET scan identifies differences in metabolism between normal and diseased tissues, and is currently being evaluated for its usefulness in detecting ovarian cancer.

X-rays of the digestive tract may be done, to determine whether a primary tumor is there rather than in the ovaries. It is not unusual

> The worst part is waiting for my tumor marker results, or the results of the CT scan or PET scan. That's the most anxiety-provoking part of life . . . waiting for these results. If the tumor markers are going up, then I'm fearful that I'm going to need more treatment. My husband and I do what we can when I'm feeling well, I don't go to a support group because I don't want to spend more time thinking about it than is necessary.
>
> —E. W.

for breast or colorectal cancers to secondarily spread to an ovary. The treatment of women with secondary cancer spread to an ovary is very different from that recommended for women with cancer that started in the ovary. It's not necessary to be hospitalized for these tests, which take about an hour or less, but some preparation—such as not eating on the morning of the test, and doing cleansing enemas the night before—may be necessary.

Blood tests may include tumor markers as well as tests to evaluate liver and kidney function. These are usually done as part of a general evaluation, when ovarian cancer is suspected.

DIAGNOSTIC SURGERY

Many benign conditions—endometriosis, ectopic pregnancy, inflammatory conditions, even hard stool in the lower intestinal tract—create a mass that can feel like a malignant tumor or look like one on an X-ray, a scan, or an ultrasound image. When a mass persists, the only way to diagnose with certainty is for a surgeon to actually retrieve tissue from the questionable area and have a pathologist examine it microscopically. (Although this surgery may be done by a general surgeon or a gynecologic surgeon, a gynecologic oncologist should be available if there is a strong suspicion of a malignancy.) A general rule of thumb among gynecologists, when they find a suspicious mass in a postmenopausal woman, is to recommend surgery to inspect the mass if it is larger than 5 centimeters (2 inches) at its greatest diameter.

Premenopausal women are more prone to developing fluid-filled cysts, which do not always warrant surgery. Serial transvaginal or abdominal (through the abdominal wall) ultrasound may answer the question of whether a mass is a benign cyst or a solid tumor that could be malignant. If it is physiologic (for example, a temporary cyst related to normal functioning of the ovary), it will disappear after a menstrual cycle or two. A laparoscopy or laparotomy is done for a persistent mass that is larger than 5 centimeters.

Laparoscopy

This technique is sometimes called "band-aid surgery," because the actual incisions are only about a quarter of an inch. However, there may be as many as four incisions. A telescopelike viewing instrument is inserted through the abdominal incision, and the surgeon peers through it to examine the magnified surface of the ovaries and the other organs in the pelvis. Samples of tissue may be retrieved through the laparoscope.

Although general anesthesia is necessary, laparoscopy can be done on an outpatient basis. After the woman regains consciousness and her vital signs are stable, she can usually return home the same day, unless other surgical procedures such as a hysterectomy were also done.

Laparotomy

This operation is done when ovarian cancer is suspected, or to confirm a diagnosis that has been made by other means. If a biopsy by laparoscopy has shown ovarian cancer, the woman will undergo a staging laparotomy. If noninvasive testing raises the suspicion of ovarian cancer, a laparoscopy will not be done. Instead, a laparotomy is performed and the surgeon extends the examination to include other organs, tissues, and lymph nodes in the area. This surgery is sometimes called *staging*, because the results of the surgeon's findings will establish the extent of the cancer—whether it is limited to an ovary or has spread to the outside surface of the ovary and, possibly, throughout the pelvis and abdomen.

The entire procedure can be accomplished through a vertical incision in the abdominal wall. General anesthesia and hospitalization are necessary because a woman's vital signs and body fluids must be monitored after a laparotomy. Recovery in the hospital, in most cases, even when a hysterectomy is necessary, requires about three to five days.

When ovarian cancer is confirmed, the surgeon will usually remove both ovaries, the cervix and uterus, and both fallopian tubes. This is called a *total hysterectomy* with *bilateral salpingo-oophorectomy* (BSO). If cancer is found to have spread beyond the ovary, the surgeon excises as much of the cancer as possible during the operation, in what is referred to as *debulking surgery*. The surgeon also examines lymph nodes throughout the pelvis and along the major blood vessels, removing many of them for further study.

When a woman has early-stage ovarian cancer and still wants to have children, it is sometimes possible to remove the diseased ovary and adjacent fallopian tube, and leave the other side intact until she has completed her family. This decision is very difficult, and much depends on how aggressive her particular type of cancer is. Consultation with a gynecologic oncologist is recommended.

TYPES OF OVARIAN CANCER

About 85 to 90 percent of cancers of the ovary arise from the outer surface, or epithelial layer, of the organ. These epithelial tumors are categorized according to the specific type of cell involved. There are four common types: nearly half of malignant epithelial ovarian tumors are *serous*, about one-fourth are *endometrioid*, and the remainder are *mucinous* and *clear cell* cancers. *Borderline tumors* or *tumors of low malignant potential* tend to be slower-growing and thus have a better prognosis than other carcinomas. Yet, they can sometimes cause death. Borderline tumors are also subclassified according to cell type as being serous, mucinous, endometrioid, or clear cell.

Less common than epithelial tumors are stromal and germ cell cancers. Because these cancers are less common, the discussion of ovarian cancer herein will refer to epithelial ovarian cancer.

STAGING

The International Federation of Gynecology and Obstetrics (FIGO) has devised a staging system that is based on an anatomic extent of the disease and on microscopic examination of the tumor and cells found elsewhere in the pelvis or abdomen.

Cancer of the ovary spreads in a fairly predictable pattern. If the cancer extends to the surface of the ovary, cells may spread to the surrounding structures—the bladder, rectum, uterus, and fallopian tubes, and the ligaments holding the ovaries in place.

STAGING FOR CANCER OF THE OVARY

FIGO System   *Description*

I Growth limited to the ovaries (one or both).

  IA Cancer limited to one ovary; no *ascites* (accumulation of fluid in the abdomen) present containing malignant cells. No tumor on the external surface of the ovary. Capsule intact (the layer of fibrous tissue surrounding the cancer is not disrupted).

  IB Cancer limited to both ovaries; no ascites present containing malignant cells. No tumor on the external surfaces. Capsule intact.

  IC Cancer limited to one or both ovaries but with one or more of the following: tumor on the surface of one or both ovaries; or with ruptured capsule(s); or with ascites containing malignant cells present; or with positive peritoneal washing.

II Cancer involving one or both ovaries, with extension to other organs in the pelvis.

  IIA Extension and/or implants to the uterus and/or tubes. No cancer in ascites or peritoneal washings.

  IIB Extension to other pelvic organs such as the bladder or rectum. No cancer cells in ascites or peritoneal washings.

  IIC Cancer involves pelvic organs as in Stage IIA or IIB, but has one or more of the following: tumor on the surface of one or both ovaries; capsule(s) ruptured; ascites containing malignant cells present; or positive peritoneal washing.

III Cancer involving one or both ovaries with peritoneal implants outside the pelvis and/or spread to retroperitoneal or inguinal lymph nodes. Implants are cancer deposits on the outer surface of organs inside the abdomen. Tumor is limited to the true pelvis but with histologically proven malignant extension to small bowel or omentum.

  IIIA Cancer grossly limited to the true pelvis but with histologically confirmed microscopic seeding on abdominal peritoneal surfaces. Cancer deposits outside the pelvis too small for the surgeon to see are found only by viewing under the microscope. No cancer spread to lymph nodes.

IIIB   Cancer of one or both ovaries with implants on abdominal peritoneal surfaces large enough to be noted by the surgeon but still smaller than 2 cm (about ¾ inch). No cancer spread to lymph nodes.
IIIC   Abdominal implants larger than 2 cm and/or spread of cancer to retroperitoneal or inguinal lymph nodes.

IV   Cancer involving one or both ovaries, with metastases to distant organs. If pleural effusion (fluid in the chest cavity) is present, there must be positive cytologic findings (cancer cells found under the microscope) to designate a case as Stage IV. Spread to the interior of abdominal organs such as the liver is considered distant metastases indicating Stage IV cancer. On the other hand, involvement limited to the outer surface of the liver is an implant and would indicate Stage III cancer.

Cells may enter the lymphatic channels and reach the lymph nodes. Cells may be carried by the fluid that circulates through the abdomen to the diaphragm and the fatty tissue covering the abdominal organs called the *omentum*. When cancer spreads to the lining of these surfaces, it causes fluid leakage as well as blockage of lymph vessels that absorb fluid, and can result in the accumulation of up to several quarts of fluid. (Bloating is a common symptom of ovarian cancer.) When cancer cells come to rest in the pelvic and abdominal cavities, they continue to multiply and form small tumors or nodules. The surgeon searches these out during *surgical staging*.

Chapter 20

Treatment of Ovarian Cancer

Treatment of any cancer has two main objectives: (1) to control the disease locally—that is, to rid the site where the cancer originates and the adjacent tissues, of all cancer cells; and (2) to destroy any cancer cells that have spread to distant areas of the body. Ovarian cancer treatment almost always involves a combination of surgery for local and regional control and chemotherapy to treat distant spread. Radiation therapy may also be recommended in some situations.

There are no set rules regarding treatment, but there are general guidelines or treatment options, depending on the stage of the cancer and the aggressiveness of the tumor cells. This chapter describes the standard options for various stages of epithelial ovarian cancer. Keep in mind that your physician will also consider your individual needs, so these treatment guidelines may be modified or rejected entirely because of factors such as your age, your desire to have children, or how near you are to the closest hospital. To obtain the best care you can, ask your doctor about any treatment option he or she recommends: Which is best for *you?* What are possible side effects? Be direct in expressing your needs and fears, but recognize that each person—and each case of cancer—is unique, and your treatment must be tailored to fit your situation and condition.

Treatment of women with early-stage cancer may be limited to removing an ovary containing a malignant tumor, while other women with more advanced cancer may require a combination of surgery, radiation, and chemotherapy. The therapy recommended to you will depend greatly on the stage of the cancer and may also be influenced by the grade of your tumor. Grade 1 (G1) is *low-grade* or *well-differentiated*, that is, closely similar to normal cells and showing extensive arrangement of cells into glands; G2 is *moderately differentiated*; and G3 is *poorly differentiated*—the cells are quite abnormal and there is very little gland formation. The *grade* of your tumor is determined by a pathologist after examining your cancer cells under a microscope.

Surgery

Surgery to remove the uterus (hysterectomy), both fallopian tubes, and ovaries (bilateral salpingo-oophorectomy), and omentum (omentectomy) is almost always the first step in treating most women with epithelial ovarian cancer. Great care is taken to avoid a rupture of the tumor capsule, which could cause further spread of cancer cells. During this operation, the surgeon will remove lymph nodes from the pelvis and from around the major blood vessels, will take fluid samples to examine for cancer cells, and will examine the abdominal organs. Sampling lymph nodes is an integral part of accurately determining the stage of the cancer, when there is no visible spread of cancer beyond the ovaries or pelvis.

Surgery cannot cure Stage III or IV ovarian cancer, but a large study completed recently showed that removing the reproductive organs or reducing the size of tumor(s) in the ovary and elsewhere in the pelvic and abdominal cavities improved survival of women with advanced ovarian cancer. The improvement is probably the result of several things. For example, chemotherapy following this *cytoreductive* or *debulking* surgery is usually more effective, especially if any deposits of tumor that remain—the *residual* cancer—are smaller than 1 cm. In general, a gynecologic oncologist tries to reduce the size of a tumor to less than 1 cm without damaging the nearby organs. However, to complete this surgery, it may be necessary to remove some of the bowel and additional lymph nodes. Debulking surgery can also help relieve symptoms in women with advanced ovarian cancer, and some researchers think it may improve immunity.

When ovarian cancer is advanced, a *second-look laparotomy* or *second-look surgery* may be done after a period of treatment is complete, to give the gynecologic oncologist an opportunity to search for residual or recurrent cancer. But this procedure is not done by all gynecologic oncologists because it has not been shown to affect survival. If it is suggested, discuss its pros and cons with your surgeon. Surgical reassessment may be considered if what the doctor finds will affect treatment decisions. The presence of residual disease is an even more significant predictor of how long a woman will remain disease-free. During this procedure, all the abdominal organs and lymph nodes in the pelvis and near the major blood vessels are examined, and samples of fluid and tissue from specific parts of the pelvic and abdominal cavities are obtained for microscopic examination. This is a major abdominal operation that requires general anesthesia, about five to seven days in the hospital, and another three to six weeks for recovery at home.

If cancer is present, additional debulking surgery, and/or chemotherapy with different drugs, some of which are still being tested in clinical trials, may be recommended. If no cancer is found, *consolidation treatment* involving more chemotherapy may still be considered because of the high risk of recurrence. However, this treatment is considered investigational.

Radiation Therapy

In selected cases, radiation therapy may be used following surgery to destroy cancer cells that have spread from the tumor into
the pelvic or abdominal cavities. It's not effective in controlling
disease that is widespread throughout the abdomen, but it can be
useful in women who have no gross residual disease, that is,
when after surgery no cancer is detected by a surgeon or by imaging studies. The radiation may be delivered to the targeted area
from outside the body *(external beam radiation)* or by infusing
the abdomen with a radioactive phosphorus solution *(intraperitoneal P-32 radiation therapy)*.

Chemotherapy

Chemotherapy is recommended after surgery in most cases of
ovarian cancer. (One possible exception is early-stage, low-grade
ovarian cancer.) The typical course is six cycles of chemotherapy.
A *cycle* is a schedule that allows regular doses of a drug, followed
by a rest period during which the body can restore its blood cells
and recover from the side effects of the dosage. Different drugs
have varying cycles; the particular cycle or schedule for your
chemotherapy will be prescribed by your oncologist. During the
course of the therapy, you will be closely monitored to assess how
your body—particularly your blood-forming cells—is handling
these powerful substances.

These drugs are usually administered intravenously in a three-
to four-week cycle, depending on the individual's blood counts.
The drugs may also be given *intraperitoneally* (directly into the
pelvic cavity).

Several classes of chemotherapy drugs may be used singly or in
combination. However, research has established that combinations of drugs that include platinum compounds such as cisplatin

or carboplatin are more effective than single agents. In the United States, combination therapy with a platinum compound and a taxane such as paclitaxel is standard initial or *first line* treatment. There are several reasons why two or more drugs work better than one. Because each drug has certain side effects, a combination of drugs allows higher dosages of chemotherapy without risking the extreme reaction that an equivalent amount of one drug would cause. Also, cancer cells do have the ability to develop a resistance to drugs; by combining drugs, the chances of resistance may be decreased.

Although ovarian cancer tends to respond to chemotherapy, the cancer cells may eventually begin to grow again. Tumor recurrence is sometimes treated with additional cycles of a platinum compound and/or taxane. In other cases, recurrence is treated with *second line* agents such as topotecan, anthracyclines (doxorubicin), gemcitabine cyclophosphamide, hexamethylmelamine, ifosfamide, etoposide, or 5-flourouracil. All of these drugs destroy cancer cells and prevent them from reproducing. They accomplish these goals by interfering in different ways with aspects of the cell division process.

Chemotherapy drugs slow the formation of healthy blood cells, which may make it necessary to temporarily suspend treatment. Recently, researchers have found that drugs called growth factors or cytolcines, which promote blood cell production by helping the bone marrow recover more quickly, can help women receiving high doses of chemotherapy avoid certain side effects. An oncologist may prescribe them if a woman's blood count gets too low or an infection occurs.

Another area of investigation involves giving very high doses of anticancer drugs, and then "rescuing" the woman from the side effects with infusions of her own *bone marrow stem cells* or *peripheral blood stem cells* (immature blood cells that may be taken from the bone marrow or removed from the bloodstream by using a special filtering process from the bloodstream). The bone marrow or peripheral blood stem cells are removed before large amounts of chemotherapy are administered and is returned to the woman (reinfused) after the high-dose treatment is complete. In that way, the side effect of suppressed blood cell production is overcome. This is an extremely high-risk, experimental procedure because, for a time, the woman is without her normal supply of blood cells and is very vulnerable to infection. It is also a costly procedure that is not available in many community hospitals and may not be covered by all health care plans. Because bone marrow/stem cell transplantation is considered experimental, a woman seeking this treatment should do so in a *clinical trial*—that is, as a participant in a formal study.

Side Effects

In addition to their effects on blood cell formation, anticancer therapies and drugs cause other problems that can seriously alter your quality of life. These effects range from nausea and vomiting during the course of therapy to temporary hair loss and premature menopause.

Should side effects become severe—for instance, the vomiting causes serious dehydration—or life-threatening—such as bone marrow suppression—the patient may have to be hospitalized.

TREATMENT BY STAGE

The following discussion refers to treatment for epithelial ovarian cancer, which is the type affecting nearly 90 percent of women with ovarian cancer.

Stages IA and IB

A total hysterectomy and removal of the ovaries and fallopian tubes (bilateral salpingo-oophorectomy or BSO) are often sufficient for controlling early-stage, low-grade ovarian cancer. Women with Stage IA or Stage IB tumors that are well or moderately differentiated have a five-year disease-free survival rate of 91 to 98 percent, which is not improved by adjuvant therapy.

A woman with a low-grade tumor who wishes to have children may choose to preserve her fertility for a few years by having removal of only the affected ovary, the fallopian tube on that side, and the omentum, plus lymph node sampling. After she has completed her family, her surgeon will operate again to remove the opposite ovary, fallopian tube, and uterus, in the hope of preventing a cancer recurrence.

Early-stage, high-grade ovarian cancer usually requires surgery and additional (adjuvant) therapy, in the form of radiation therapy or systemic or intraperitoneal chemotherapy.

Stage IC

The standard surgery is to remove the uterus, both ovaries, both fallopian tubes, and samples of lymph nodes and omentum. Chemotherapy and possibly intraperitoneal radiation therapy are used afterward for the majority of women. The 5-year survival rate is about 90 percent.

Stage II

After the uterus, both ovaries, both fallopian tubes, lymph node samples, and part of the omentum are surgically removed, and as much tumor as possible is removed from other tissues (debulking surgery), patients will receive chemotherapy and, more rarely, radiation therapy regardless of the grade of the cancer. The five-year survival rate for Stage II is about 80 percent.

Stages III and IV

Initial surgical treatment is usually the same as for Stage II. As explained in the section on surgery for ovarian cancer, a *second-look laparotomy* may be recommended to determine whether additional debulking surgery, radiation therapy, or chemotherapy is needed.

If no residual cancer is found, consolidation treatment with systemic chemotherapy or with intraperitoneal (given directly into the pelvic and abdominal cavity), chemotherapy or radioactive phosphorous may be recommended, but this treatment is considered investigational.

If only small tumor deposits are found during second-look surgery, treatment options include more systemic or intraperitoneal chemotherapy or intraperitoneal or external beam radiation therapy.

When large tumor deposits are found by second-look surgery, the outlook is usually poor. Depending on a woman's general medical condition and preferences, participation in a clinical trial of new treatments may be worthwhile or she may wish to limit treatment to those focused on relieving symptoms.

The five-year survival rates for Stages III and IV are 15 to 20 percent, and less than 5 percent, respectively.

Recurrent Ovarian Cancer

Treatment is based on the amount of cancer present, how much time has elapsed between initial treatment and recurrence, the woman's initial treatment, and the stage of her cancer when it was diagnosed. Treatment options include debulking surgery, chemotherapy, and rarely, radiation therapy.

Tumors of Low Malignant Potential

Tumors of low malignant potential (borderline tumors) are slow growing cancers and are treated surgically, the same way as fully malignant tumors of the same stage. The difference in their treatment is that chemotherapy and radiation therapy are not recommended for adjuvant (after surgery) therapy of borderline tumors. These treatments have not been found to improve the likelihood of cure or to extend survival.

EXPERIMENTAL THERAPY

Surgery alone is never sufficient to treat advanced ovarian cancer, beyond Stage IC. By definition, advanced disease is characterized by spread of the cancer within the pelvis and abdomen and perhaps to distant sites. Women with advanced cancer are often encouraged to enter clinical trials in which they may be given new drugs or new combinations of standard therapies that have not yet been proven effective.

A number of new approaches to ovarian cancer are under study, including high-dose chemotherapy using five to ten times the usual amount of anticancer drugs, treatment with immunological agents designed to boost the body's own natural resistance to cancer, and gene therapy, in which genes are introduced into the cancer cells to alter their behavior.

To learn about clinical trials you might enter, ask your oncologist and/or contact the National Cancer Institute (800-4-CANCER).

Chapter 21

Life after Cancer

Although the treatment of your cancer is behind you—you've recovered from the surgery, the many cycles of chemotherapy are complete, the daily visits for radiation therapy are finally over—don't be surprised that your concerns about the disease remain. Naturally, you will still worry: Will the cancer come back? Did the treatment work? Will I ever feel like my old self again? Your visits to the oncologist for checkups and monitoring continually remind you that the cancer might recur. Also, you may have to deal with lasting side effects of the therapy. Surgery may have compromised your usual activities in some way, forcing you to cope with permanent changes and to make certain emotional and physical adjustments in your life. For all these reasons—and because there is a possibility that the cancer will recur—cancer is now considered by many experts to be a chronic disease. But, as many cancer survivors will attest, you can live with cancer in a satisfying and successful way. Along with the physical care you may still require and the need for periodic monitoring, the cancer experience is now part of your life.

CHECKUPS

The hope and the probability that your cancer is cured are constantly being tested with checkups. These are usually more frequent in the months immediately following treatment. Gradually, as the months and years go by, the intervals between visits to the oncologist become longer and longer. Initially, going for a checkup may be especially anxiety-provoking; people respond in various ways to that stress. Understanding what is being done, and why, may give you some control over your anxiety. Rather than thinking of the checkup as a test that you will either pass or fail, view it as a way of caring for yourself on a routine basis. Early detection of the original cancer increases the likelihood of more quality time and the chance of a cure. Early detection of any spread or recurrence often improves your chances of controlling it.

The first five years after treatment may be the most challenging: If the cancer is going to come back, it will most likely happen during this period. In general, when cancer spreads or recurs, it does so in predictable sites, so your checkups will be focused on specific areas. Breast cancer, for example, may recur in the same breast after lumpectomy, in the mastectomy scar, or in the lymph nodes under the arm. The most common distant sites of breast cancer recurrence are the bones, lungs, soft tissue, and liver. Follow-up physical exams and tests are geared toward detection of cancer recurrence in the breast and lymph nodes, or the spread of cancer to those specific distant sites.

Detecting cancer recurrence is not the only reason for your follow-up visits. Your physician also wants to make sure that you are recovering well, with maximum relief from any lingering side effects of the cancer treatment, and that you are maintaining good health in general. Most physicians are as concerned about your emotional recovery as they are about your physical healing, so if any concerns, fears, or other difficulties are on your mind, bring them up during these visits with your doctor.

After you have completed your treatment—whether it's surgery, radiation therapy, and/or chemotherapy—your primary physician will ask you to return regularly so he or she can perform a general physical checkup. The intervals at which these checkups take place vary. (See "Screening Tests," in Chapter 1, for specific guidelines.)

FOLLOW-UP TESTING

Depending on the stage of your cancer at the time of diagnosis, and the appearance of any symptoms, your oncologist may recommend a chest X-ray; special scans, such as a bone scan; and certain blood tests. There is no evidence that having these tests routinely—that is, if you have no symptoms of recurrence—is of any value in terms of increasing survival. However, after treatment for ovarian cancer, for example, a blood test for the antigen CA-125 is done periodically. The CA-125 test is not foolproof for detecting cancer recurrence, but it is the best blood test currently available.

Pap Test and Pelvic Examination

The American Cancer Society has specific guidelines for when and how often women without symptoms, risk factors, or previous reproductive system cancer should have a pelvic examination and Pap smear. Women who have been treated for cervical intraepithelial neoplasia or cancer of the cervix typically have these tests more often than annually for several years.

In the past, some doctors that treated women for breast cancer with tamoxifen have done routine endometerial biopsy specimens

> You're always living on a picket fence. Every time I go to my doctor, I
> go with my fingers crossed. The last time I was there, she said, "You're
> cancer-free!" That's fine. I walked out very happy. The only problem is
> the radiation burned my bladder, now that's the problem today.
>
> —M. S.

to rule out hyperplasia or cancer. This is now felt to be unnecessary, but it is very important that these women report any abnormal vaginal bleeding, which indicates that a biopsy is needed.

Mammography

If you have had a lumpectomy, a mammogram will be done six
months after completing radiation therapy, and at least once a
year afterward.

Both the American College of Radiology and the American
Cancer Society recommend mammography of the opposite breast
annually, or more often if any abnormalities are noted. (If you
have had a lumpectomy, you should have a mammogram of both
breasts.) The risk of cancer is about the same for the treated and
the untreated breast.

SCREENING GUIDELINES FOR OTHER SYSTEMS

The American Cancer Society has recommended several tests to
be done routinely on people who have no symptoms or health
problems. With all the attention given to looking for any recurrence of your breast, cervix, endometrial, or ovarian cancer, it's
important that you not overlook screening tests for cancer of other

systems unless your doctors recommend that it is fine to do so. (See "Screening Tests," in Chapter 1.)

Self-exams should be a routine part of your health care. These include skin self-exam—a visual examination of your entire body, front and back, for unusual skin growths, pigmented spots, and sores. The American Cancer Society does not have a specific recommendation for frequency, but the Skin Cancer Foundation advises a skin-exam every three months, and a physician's examination of your skin every year. Some doctors and dentists recommend examining your mouth and tongue for abnormalities, too, especially if you are or have been a smoker.

WHEN TO CALL YOUR DOCTOR

It's natural to become alarmed when physical ailments or symptoms appear, but knowing the conditions that are real health concerns should keep your reactions under informed control. Let your doctor know if you experience a continuing loss of appetite or of weight; pain in your back, shoulders, lower back, or pelvis; headaches; dizziness; blurred vision; coughing or hoarseness; or digestive problems. Call your doctor if you have any changes in your menstrual periods or any unusual vaginal bleeding.

If you notice any changes or problems—such as pain, redness, swelling, lumps, or thickening—in the breast that was operated on or in the scar, call your doctor.

LIFE AS A CANCER SURVIVOR

Today, more women are cancer survivors than ever before, and survival rates are steadily increasing. Surviving cancer means not only that the disease is under control but that you are able to participate in your family life and community.

Returning to Work and Life

How soon you return to work following cancer treatment varies, of course, according to the stage of your illness and the treatment required. Many women with early-stage breast cancer, for example, return to work within days of having had a lumpectomy, and they continue working while they are receiving daily radiation therapy. But if you've had a mastectomy for breast cancer or a hysterectomy for cervical, endometrial, or ovarian cancer, your physical recovery will take some time and returning to your previous life may demand some temporary adjustment. For instance, you may find that you tire more easily. If your job requires physical strength or endurance (if, say, you must lift heavy things or you are on your feet much of the time), you may need to wait until you've regained your strength to return to the same job.

It's natural to be concerned about how others will respond to you. In fact, you may choose not to share the fact that you've been treated for cancer with anyone beyond your closest friends and family. Or, you may believe that being open and offering coworkers and neighbors a direct if brief explanation of your condition is the best approach. Only you can decide what suits your personality, your privacy needs, and your employment situation.

Your rights are protected by law, however, and it is illegal for your employer to treat you differently because you have been treated for cancer. This is one area where myths abound. The truth is that people with cancer are often as productive as they were before they were diagnosed. According to a Metropolitan Life Insurance Company study, cancer survivors have the same job turnover rate as those who had no such history, and their absentee rate is only slightly higher. Some studies have shown that people with cancer have fewer sick days than their coworkers. Nevertheless, employers and coworkers can make unfair assumptions, and there have been cases of discrimination. Your local American Cancer Society office can give you information about your employment rights if you have any concerns about the attitude of those for whom you work.

If you have any doubts about what you can do, how hard you can work, how you can manage your job, or your job security, discuss those concerns with your physician. Social workers can be of great assistance, too. They counsel many women with cancer and have experience helping people cope in a variety of situations and professions. Ask your primary health care provider for a reference at your community's Department of Social Services.

Joining a support group may also be useful (see the Resources section that follows this chapter). A support group is also a place where you can share how you're learning to live with cancer and thereby help others, which is tremendously satisfying. Organizations of cancer survivors who have faced a situation similar to yours not only offer support and encouragement but also keep you up-to-date on new treatments and developments and on political, legal, and health care situations. Being informed can diminish many of the fears that arise during this phase of your recovery.

Lifestyle Change

There is no proof that changing your diet, exercising more, quitting smoking, and practicing stress reduction techniques will prevent a recurrence, but all of these measures—and other steps you can take to maintain a healthy lifestyle—are likely to enhance your recovery from cancer treatment and improve the quality of your life.

> Sitting in the hospital support group really depressed me. The women were much older than me. That was the depressing part . . . being the youngest one. I just felt like, "Why me?"
>
> —P. S.

You may find that returning to your "normal" life may take some time, but taking one step at a time toward that goal will naturally bring you closer to it. For example, rather than sitting down to three meals a day, as you may have before cancer treatment, eating small meals as many as six or more times a day may provide you with the nourishment you need to regain your strength and appetite. Walking just a few minutes several times a day, gradually increasing the time and distance week by week, will improve the ability of your lungs to take in more and more oxygen and strengthen your heart and other muscles. Cancer survivors and others recovering from serious surgery often say that regular exercise helps them feel more energetic. Working out with weights— beginning with small weights and gradually increasing the amount—also helps build muscle. Regular stretching improves flexibility, which is particularly important if you have been confined to bed or your movement has been limited. It may be easier to exercise regularly if you are part of a group such as Encore, which is organized by the YWCA specifically for cancer survivors.

Sexuality and Intimacy

The health of your relationship and the degree of sexual satisfaction you experienced before your cancer was diagnosed are far more important predictors of your sexual satisfaction after cancer treatment than the extent of your surgery. Most women who have a modified radical mastectomy, for instance, cope well with the surgery and the physical change in their body, and they don't report a change in the frequency of sexual activity. According to one study, women who were receiving chemotherapy reported less sexual activity, but their ability to have an orgasm was not affected.

There is no evidence to support the belief that a hysterectomy affects a woman's ability to become sexually aroused or to have an orgasm. However, when the ovaries are removed and menopause occurs, vaginal dryness may occur. Because estrogen replacement therapy, which would help resolve this side effect, may not be advised, it may be necessary to use lubricants specifically designed for this problem. For some women, intravaginal estrogen is allowed. The issue of estrogen replacement in survivors of breast and reproductive system cancer is complex and controversial, and decisions may be influenced by a woman's specific medical situation. If you have any questions, ask all of your doctors for their view of this issue.

Women with advanced cancer that has required removal of all pelvic organs—including the vagina—may or may not have reconstructive surgery, but, in either case, working with a sex therapist to learn ways to experience pleasurable sexual activity may be very helpful.

Some women have problems with their self-image. They find it difficult to adjust, and they may become depressed, which, of course, affects their sexuality. Take into account your own feelings about your body image and your sexuality when you are making treatment decisions. Surgery for breast cancer is physically obvious; gynecologic surgery is not, except for the most advanced stages of cancer. Among women undergoing breast surgery, those who have breast-conserving treatment (BCT) may have more positive feelings about their body than those who have a mastectomy.

If you believe your physical appearance significantly affects your sexual identity, and a mastectomy is your only choice, then immediate breast reconstruction is a desirable option.

Unfortunately, studies have not been completed to evaluate the specifics of sexual satisfaction. For instance, although frequency of sexual activity and the ability to have an orgasm are important measures of a satisfying sex life, they are only two aspects of the many dimensions of sexual function.

Psychologists and psychiatric social workers who are members of treatment teams have learned the importance of talking with women and their partners about how the cancer treatment affects their emotional and sexual responses. A professional can open up a dialogue *between the couple* about topics that may be difficult for them to discuss, and, in that context, can suggest sexual techniques and answer questions, such as whether a scar can be touched, how nudity can be more comfortable, which sexual positions are best during healing, and what lubricants can be used to counter the dryness related to surgery-induced or chemotherapy-induced menopause.

Women who do not have partners bring additional issues to a counselor, such as how and when should they tell someone they're dating about their history of cancer? A support group that includes single women can be especially helpful.

For the majority of women, physical and psychological adjustment will be needed, but the love they share with their partner, and their desire to be intimate, can endure beyond their cancer treatment and may grow deeper because of it.

Quality of Life

From the moment you heard your diagnosis of cancer, your life has been a barrage of tests, procedures, information gathering, and waiting. Much of that is now behind you; your mind and body are moving through a gradual process of repair. For some women, the healing will be complete and uneventful; for others, the battle against cancer will continue. Whichever group you belong to, the best thing you can do for yourself—and those close to you—is to maintain the highest quality of life you can. For every cancer survivor, exactly how to achieve that goal will be different.

Surprisingly, some cancer survivors describe how their life was changed for the better after their diagnosis. They valued life and their relationships with other people more highly. Perhaps knowing how precious life is prompted them to switch careers, alter their lifestyle, and take an active role in deepening their relationship to someone close to them.

Some women will need help in understanding their own reactions to their illness and being able to effectively meet the many challenges confronting them. Time, the encouragement of family, and perhaps the directness of a support group may be needed. Cancer survivors—like anyone who has been traumatized by some life event—may occasionally feel depressed. Psychotherapy and/or medical treatment for depression might be considered. Some women find spiritual guidance especially helpful.

Many of the resources listed in the next section can provide you with referrals and information on support services. Now that people share more openly their experiences with cancer, you may find groups and services as near as your community center, a local church, and, of course, the hospital where you were treated. Although the numbers of women facing cancer are finally beginning to level, it may help you to know that there is always a cancer survivor who would be willing to share her story and support you in your battle.

Clinical Trials

During your course of your cancer treatment, your doctor may suggest that you take part in a clinical trial. Clinical trials are studies of new treatments in patients that are undertaken to compare their effectiveness, risks and side effects with those of standard treatments. All trials provide at least the current standard for treatment. These studies are begun only after laboratory studies strongly suggest that the new treatment may indeed be of value to patients. However, there are some risks. No one knows in advance whether the treatment will work and exactly what side effects may occur.

As with any standard cancer treatment, clinical trials involve informed consent—your doctors and nurses will explain details of the treatment being tested and give you a form to read and sign, indicating your understanding and your desire to take part. Participation in any clinical trial is completely voluntary. Even after signing the consent form and after the trial begins, you are free to leave the study at any time. Taking part in clinical trials may help you directly, or may help find better cancer treatments in the future.

You can find out about clinical trials from your cancer care team. Don't hesitate to ask questions about the study such as:

What is the purpose of the study?

What kinds of tests and treatments are involved?

What are the standard treatment options and their advantages and disadvantages?

What side effects are most likely to occur?

How long will the study last?

Will I have to be hospitalized? If so, how often and for how long?

Will the study cost me anything? Will any of the treatments be free?

If I am harmed as a result of the research, what treatment would I be entitled to?

What type of long-term follow-up care is part of the study?

You can get a list of current clinical trials by calling the National Cancer Institute's Cancer Information Service toll free at 800-4-CANCER. Information about clinical trials of breast cancer treatment is available from the National Alliance of Breast Cancer Organizations.

Resources

AMERICAN CANCER SOCIETY PUBLICATIONS

The following publications are available through the American Cancer Society. Call 800-ACS-2345 to request a free copy.

A Significant Journey (video)
   Narrated by a breast cancer survivor and her husband. It chronicles the passage from diagnosis to recovery and the ways that breast cancer affects a loving relationship.

After Diagnosis: A Guide for Patients
   Provides general information patients and their families need to know after a cancer diagnosis. Describes the people and services that are available to help cope with cancer.

Americans with Disabilities Act
   Looks at the definition of disability and answers questions about how the law applies to people with cancer in the workplace.

Breast Cancer Questions and Answers
   Answers nine of the most common and important questions about breast cancer. Also available in Spanish.

Breast Reconstruction after Mastectomy

Describes the various types of breast reconstruction choices available to women after a mastectomy. Includes illustrations as well as information on planning and preparing for surgery. Also available in Spanish.

Caring for the Patient with Cancer at Home

Provides cancer patients and their families with information about cancer and cancer treatment. Over 50 topics cover signs and symptoms, what to look for, and when to call the doctor.

Get Relief from Cancer Pain

Produced jointly with the National Cancer Institute. Easy to read pamphlet helps to increase patient awareness of the importance of treating cancer pain. Emphasizes the patient's right to pain control and encourages them to talk to their doctors and nurses about getting adequate pain relief. Also available in Spanish.

Listen with Your Heart

Assists friends and family members in understanding the patient's needs and feelings.

Sexuality and Cancer—For the Woman Who Has Cancer and Her Partner

Offers in-depth information about cancer and sexuality in the areas that most concern the woman with cancer and her partner.

Talking with Your Doctor

Assists patients in building a good working relationship with their doctors through effective communication.

tlc Magalog

For women with breast cancer, breast cancer survivors and women who are experiencing hair loss due to cancer treatment.

Offers a wide variety of products, including hats and turbans, mastectomy bras, breast forms and silicone prostheses. Also features useful information for cancer survivors.

Understanding Chemotherapy
    Answers many questions about this method of cancer treatment.

Understanding Radiation Therapy
    Answers questions about radiation therapy.

ADDITIONAL READING

(Inclusion on this list does not imply endorsement by the American Cancer Society)

A *Cancer Survivor's Almanac: Charting Your Journey.* Edited by Barbara Hoffman, JD. National Coalition for Cancer Survivorship. New York: Chronimed Publishing, 1996.
Capossela, Cappy, and Sheila Warnock. *Share the Care: How to Organize a Group for Someone Who Is Seriously Ill.* New York: Simon & Schuster, 1995.
Hirshaut, Yashar and Peter Pressman. *Breast Cancer: The Complete Guide.* New York: Bantam, 1996.
Lange, Vladimir. *Be a Survivor: Your Guide to Breast Cancer Treatment* (book, video and CD-ROM). Los Angeles: Lange Productions, 1998.
Murphy, G. P., L. P. Morris, and D. Lange. *Informed Decisions: The Complete Book of Cancer Diagnosis, Treatment, and Recovery.* New York: Viking, 1997.
A *Portrait of Breast Cancer: Expressions in Words and Art.* American Cancer Society—edited by William D. Smith, Ph.D. (a collection of essays and art created by those who have

experienced breast cancer). Atlanta: American Cancer Society, 1997.

Robinson, Rebecca Y., and Jeanne A. Petrek. A *Step-by-Step Guide to Dealing with Your Breast Cancer*. New York: Carol Publishing Group, 1996.

Runowicz, Carolyn D., and D. Haupt. *To Be Alive: A Woman's Guide to a Full Life after Cancer*. New York: Henry Holt & Co., 1996.

Schover, Leslie R. *Sexuality and Fertility after Cancer*. New York: John Wiley & Sons, Inc., 1997.

The listings in the following section are gathered under the following headings, which are arranged in alphabetical order:

	Page
American Cancer Society	249
Breast Cancer Resources	250
Counseling and Support Groups	251
Family Support	254
General Information on Cancer	255
Gynecologic Cancers	257
Home Health Care	260
Hospice and Supportive Services	261
Money and Insurance	263
Pain Management	263
YWCA	264

AMERICAN CANCER SOCIETY

I Can Cope

The American Cancer Society is the nationwide voluntary health organization dedicated to eliminating cancer as a major health problem by preventing cancer, saving lives from cancer, and diminishing suffering from cancer through research, education, and services.

For detailed information about cancer and cancer-related topics, you can call 800-ACS-2345. The service is available 24 hours a day, 7 days a week. Or visit the ACS web site at www.cancer.org.

In addition, programs such as Reach to Recovery, Look Good, Feel Better, and I Can Cope may be available in your area. Call the 800 number for more information about these or other local programs.

Look Good, Feel Better
800-395-LOOK (800-395-5665)
A free program dedicated to teaching women with cancer how to restore a healthy appearance and self-image during chemotherapy or radiation therapy.

Reach to Recovery
800-ACS-2345 (800-227-2345)
Reach to Recovery is an ACS visitation program for women and their families who have a personal concern about breast cancer. Trained volunteers who have experienced breast cancer themselves provide information and support. An early component of the program provides support to women who have a suspicious lump or mammogram or who have just received a breast cancer diagnosis but have not begun treatment. Reach to Recovery volunteers can help a woman by giving her an opportunity to express her feelings, verbalize her fears and concerns, and ask questions of someone who is impartial and objective.

BREAST CANCER RESOURCES

American Society of Plastic and Reconstructive Surgeons
(ASPRS)
444 East Algonquin Road
Arlington Heights, IL 60005
800-635-0635 (24-hour referral service an option)
708-228-9900
Fax: 708-228-0117
www.plasticsurgery.org
*Offers brochures on breast reconstruction. May supply the names
of board-certified plastic surgeons in your area who are ASPRS
members. Will also verify whether your surgeon is board-certified.*

National Alliance of Breast Cancer Organizations
9 E. 37th Street, 10th Floor
New York, NY 10016
800-719-9154
www.nabco.org
*National Alliance of Breast Cancer Organizations (NABCO), a
network of 370 breast cancer organizations, provides information,
assistance and referral to anyone with questions about breast cancer, and acts as a voice for the interests and concerns of breast cancer survivors and women at risk.*

National Lymphedema Network
2211 Post Street, Suite 404
San Francisco, CA 94115
800-541-3259
415-921-2911
Fax: 415-921-4284
www.hooked.net/~lymphnet
*Offers information and education about lymphedema, referrals to
medical and therapeutic treatment centers, and information on lo-
cating or establishing support groups. Quarterly newsletter lists
local support groups.*

Susan G. Komen Breast Cancer Foundation
5005 LBJ Freeway, Suite 370
Dallas, TX 75240
800-462-9273
Fax: 972-855-1640
www.breastcancerinfo.com
Volunteer organization that assists women in dealing with breast cancer by raising funds for screening centers, legislative advocacy, education, preclinical laboratory research, and clinical research. The primary fund-raising event is "Race for the Cure."

Y-ME National Breast Cancer Organization
212 West Van Buren
Chicago, IL 60607
800-221-2141
Spanish: 800-986-9505
24-hour hotline (emergency only): 312-926-8228
Fax: 312-986-0020
www.y-me.org
Serves women with breast cancer, and their families and friends, through a national hotline, open-door groups, and early-detection workshops. Offers peer support programs featuring breast cancer survivors and their spouses, for those currently affected by breast cancer.

COUNSELING AND SUPPORT GROUPS

AMC Cancer Research Center and Hospital
1600 Pierce Street
Denver, CO 80214
800-321-1557
Toll-free line provides up-to-date facts about cancer and personal assistance from counselors trained in dealing with the fear,

confusion, conflicts, and other problems associated with cancer.
For information on support groups, call 303-239-3424.

Cancer Care, Inc.
1180 Avenue of the Americas
New York, NY 10036
800-813-HOPE (800-813-4673) (counseling line)
212-221-3300
Fax: 212-719-0263
www.cancercareinc.org
Cancer Care is a national, nonprofit organization that helps people
with cancer, their families, and professional caregivers. Through
one-to-one counseling, specialized support groups, educational pro-
grams, and telephone contact, Cancer Care provides support, guid-
ance, information, and referral free of charge.

Cancervive
6500 Wilshire Boulevard, Suite 500
Los Angeles, CA 90048
310-203-9232
Offers telephone counseling, referrals, and education to people
with cancer.

Make Today Count
Mid-America Cancer Center
1235 East Cherokee
Springfield, MO 65804-2263
800-432-2273
417-885-2273
Fax: 417-888-7426
Support organization for people affected by cancer or other life-
threatening illness; outreach includes families and health care
professionals.

The Mautner Project for Lesbians with Cancer
1707 L Street NW, Suite 1060
Washington, DC 20036
202-332-5536
Fax: 202-265-6854
www.mautnerproject.org
Provides education, information, and advocacy for health issues relating to lesbians with cancer and their families.

National Coalition for Cancer Survivorship (NCCS)
1010 Wayne Avenue, Fifth Floor
Silver Spring, MD 20910
888-937-6227
301-650-8868
www.cansearch.org
Serves as a clearinghouse for information, publications, and programs for organizations that work on survivorship issues. Promotes study of problems and potentials of survivorship, and advocates interests of cancer survivors to secure their rights and combat prejudice.

National Women's Health Information Center (NWHIC)
200 Independence Avenue, SW-Room 712E
Washington, DC 20201
800-994-WOMAN or 800-994-9662—Also has Spanish speaking health information specialists.
Fax: 301-961-0280
www.4woman.org
Federal government information referral service for women's health sponsored by the U.S. Department of Health and Human Services—Public Health Service's Office on Women's Health. Answers questions on women's health by information on organizations and publications. Main purpose of the NWHIC is an information referral service.

Information includes databases on federal and private organizations, federal government publications, resources, current news articles and events, and reference materials. Limited number of Spanish publications available. Business hours are 10:00 A.M.–6:00 P.M. EST, Monday–Friday.

The Wellness Community—National
2716 Ocean Park Boulevard, Suite 1040
Santa Monica, CA 90405-5211
310-314-2555
Fax: 310-314-7586
Offers support to people with cancer and their families at no charge, as an adjunct to conventional medical treatment in thirteen U.S. cities. Support groups are led by licensed psychotherapists.

FAMILY SUPPORT

Bone Marrow Transplant Family Support Network
P.O. Box 845
Avon, CT 06001
800-826-9376
Telephone support network for bone marrow transplant patients and their families.

National Association of Hospital Hospitality Houses, Inc.
4915 Auburn Avenue, Suite 303
Bethesda, MD 20814
800-542-9730
Fax: 301-961-3094
www.visit-usa.com
This is a referral hotline for temporary low-cost (or no-cost) lodging for patients and their caregivers seeking medical treatment outside their own community. Services vary from facility to facility.

National Family Caregivers Association
9621 East Bexhill Drive
Kensington, MD 20895
800-896-3650
301-942-6430
Fax: 301-942-2303
www.nfcacares.org
*Provides research, education, support, advocacy, and respite care to
caregivers.*

Well Spouse Foundation
610 Lexington Avenue, Suite 814
New York, NY 10022-6005
800-838-0879
212-644-1241
Fax: 212-644-1338
*Provides emotional support for spouses/partners who are caregivers
of the chronically ill. Referrals to local support groups throughout
the country.*

GENERAL INFORMATION ON CANCER

Food and Drug Administration
Office of Consumer Affairs
HFE-88
5600 Fishers Lane
Rockville, MD 20857
Breast Implant Information Hotline
800-532-4440
*Women considering or recovering from breast reconstruction using
implants can obtain an information package.*

Hereditary Cancer Institute
Creighton University
2500 California Plaza
Omaha, NE 68178
402-280-2942
Fax: 402-280-1734
Research of hereditary colon, breast, ovarian, and pancreatic cancer and malignant melanoma in families. Services include screening recommendations and genetic testing of eligible families.

National Cancer Institute
Cancer Information Service
800-4-CANCER (800-422-6237)
www.cancernet.nci.nih.gov
Offers free publications, lists FDA-certified mammography centers, and has cancer information specialists who will tell you where clinical trials are taking place and answer your questions in English or Spanish.

National Library of Medicine
8600 Rockville Pike
Bethesda, MD 20894
800-638-8480
800-272-4787 (MEDLARS)
www.nlm.nih.gov/databases/freemedl.html
MEDLARS is the online database of National Library of Medicine.

U.S. Public Health Services Offices of Women's Health
200 Independence Avenue, SW, room 73013
Washington, DC 20201
www.4women.gov
Provides national leadership in advancing women's health through public policy, research, service delivery, and education.

GYNECOLOGIC CANCERS

Conversations! The Newsletter for Those Fighting Ovarian Cancer
P.O. Box 79114
Amarillo, TX 79114
806-355-2565
Fax: 806-467-9757
www.ovarian-news.com
Monthly newsletter reports on treatment options, clinical trials, coping skills, and early detection strategies. Networking services to match women in similar circumstances provided.

Diethylestilbestrol (DES)
DES Action USA
1615 Broadway, Suite 510
Oakland, CA 94612
800-DES-9288 (800-337-9288)
800-DES-NEWS (NY) (800-337-6397)
Fax: 510-465-4815
www.desaction.org
Dedicated to informing women about DES and helping DES-exposed women. Publishes a quarterly newsletter, The DES Action Voice, *and many publications on DES exposure. Provides link among DES-exposed women, researchers, and the medical community.*

DES Cancer Network
P.O. Box 10185
Rochester, NY 14610
716-473-6119
800-DES-NET4 (800-337-6384)
Fax: 716-473-4979

A network for women and men exposed to DES, with a special focus on cancer. Offers referrals, education, research advocacy, an annual conference for cancer survivors, and a newsletter.

Gilda Radner Familial Ovarian Cancer Registry
Roswell Park Cancer Institute
Elm and Carlton Streets
Buffalo, NY 14263
800-682-7426
Fax: 716-845-7608
www.ovariancancer.com
A registry for women with two or more first-degree relatives with ovarian cancer. Source of public education and information regarding diagnostic tests, risk factors, and warning signs.

Gilda's Club
195 West Houston Street
New York, NY 10014
212-647-9700
Provides a place where women with cancer, and their families and friends, join with others to build social and emotional support as a supplement to medical care. Free of charge.

Gynecologic Cancer Foundation
401 North Michigan Avenue
Chicago, IL 60611
800-444-4441
312-644-6610
312-527-6640
www.sgo.org and www.wcn.org
Founded by physician members of the Society of Gynecologic Oncologists to support philanthropic programs that reduce the impact of gynecologic cancers on the health of women and their families. Offers a physician referral service and information about gynecologic cancers.

Hysterectomy Educational Resources and Services (HERS)
422 Bryn Mawr Avenue
Bala Cynwyd, PA 19004
610-667-7757
Fax: 610-667-8096
The Hysterectomy Educational Resources and Services Foundation is a nonprofit organization that provides information to the general public about hysterectomy (surgical removal of the uterus) and oophorectomy (removal of the ovaries). They provide telephone counseling and support services to women who are scheduled to have or who recently have had a hysterectomy.

National Ovarian Cancer Coalition, Inc.
P.O. Box 4472
Boca Raton, FL 33429
1-888-OVARIAN (1-888-682-7426)
561-393-3220
Fax: 561-361-8804
www.ovarian.org
National Ovarian Cancer Coalition (NOCC) is a nonprofit organization founded by ovarian cancer survivors in April 1995. There are no fees or dues for membership. Its mission is to save women's lives by raising awareness about ovarian cancer and to promote education regarding all the facts, issues, and problems surrounding ovarian cancer throughout the general population and medical community.

Services include patient support groups, NOCC state chapters, a physician referral database of 400 gynecologic oncologists, physician task force, public awareness campaign, newsletter and community lectures and symposiums. Other services include on-line chat groups, quilt projects, medical facts, news and updates, and an experts forum.

Ovarian Cancer National Alliance
P.O. Box 33107
Washington, DC 20033
202-452-5910
Fax: 202-530-2901
www.ovariancancer.org
*National umbrella works to increase public and professional un-
derstanding of ovarian cancer, public policy and advocacy for
more effective diagnosis and treatments. Materials include awareness information and national public policy issue papers.*

*Ovarian Plus International: Gynecological Cancer Prevention
Quarterly*
P.O. Box 498
Paauilo, HI 96776
808-776-1696
www.monitor.net/ovarian
*Newsletter with information about research, diagnosis, and treat-
ment for ovarian and other gynecological cancers.*

HOME HEALTH CARE

National Association for Home Care
228 7th Street, SE
Washington, DC 20003
202-547-7424
Fax: 202-547-3540
www.nahc.org
*Provides information and referral to state associations of licensed
home health agencies. Please request information in writing.*

Visiting Nurse Association of America (VNAA)
National Office
3801 East Florida Avenue, Suite 900
Denver, CO 80210
800-426-2547
303-753-0218
Fax: 303-753-0258
www.vnaa.org
Organization of visiting nurse associations. Members provide nursing and assistance with bathing, dressing, and eating.

HOSPICE AND SUPPORTIVE SERVICES

Choice in Dying
1035 30th Street NW
Washington, DC 20007
800-989-WILL (800-989-9455)
www.choices.org
Concerned with protecting the rights and serving the needs of people who are dying of any illness, and their families. Distributes free information on drafting a living will and a power of attorney, and offers a free counseling service on end-of-life issues.

Foundation for Hospice and Home Care
228 7th Street NE
Washington, DC 20003
202-547-7424
Fax: 202-547-3540
www.nahc.org
Broad array of programs to serve the dying, disabled, and disadvantaged.

Hospice Association of America
228 7th Street, SE
Washington, DC 20003
202-546-4759
Membership organization for all hospices; offers addresses of local hospice organizations.

Hospice Education Institute
(HOSPICELINK)
190 Westbrook Road
Essex, CT 06426-0713
800-331-1620
Provides general information about hospice care and referrals to local hospices throughout the country.

National Hospice Organization
1901 North Moore Street, Suite 901
Arlington, VA 22209
800-658-8898
Fax: 703-525-5762
www.nho.org
Provides printed information on hospices and makes referrals to local hospices providing services to terminally ill patients. Publishes a guide to the nation's hospices.

National Institute for Jewish Hospices
8723 Alden Drive, Suite 219
Los Angeles, CA 90048
310-854-3036
213-HOSPICE (213-476-7423)
800-446-4448
Fax: 310-854-5683 (call before faxing)
Provides hospice care, counseling, and referrals with a Jewish perspective.

MONEY AND INSURANCE

Breast Cancer Screening—Medicare Coverage
Medicare provides coverage for annual screening mammography for women over age 39. The deductible is waived for mammography. In addition to the monthly premium charged to individuals enrolled in Medicare's Part B, an annual deductible of $100 is required, and a 20 percent coinsurance or copayment is required as a sharing of the expense above the deductible. Medicare pays 80 percent of the Medicare-approved charge after the $100 deductible is satisfied.

PAIN MANAGEMENT

American Academy of Pain Medicine
4700 West Lake Avenue
Glenville, IL 60025
847-375-4731
Fax: 847-375-4777
www.painmed.org
Supports care to people suffering with pain, through research, the education and training of physicians, and the advancement of the specialty of pain medicine. Provides information regarding specific pain medications.

National Chronic Pain Outreach Association
7979 Old Georgetown Road, Suite 100
Bethesda, MD 20814-2429
301-652-4948
Fax: 301-907-0745
Educates patients, health care professionals, and the public about chronic pain and its treatment.

YWCA

Encore Plus Program of the YWCA
Office of Women's Health Initiatives
624 Ninth Street NW, Third Floor
Washington, DC 20001
800-953-7587
202-628-3636
Fax: 202-783-7123
www.ywca.org
This community-based program targets medically underserved women in need of breast and cervical cancer screening and support services. Provides women treated for and recovering from breast cancer with a combined support group and exercise program.

Index

A

abdominal pain, 10–11

ablative procedures, cervical cancer, 165

abnormal cells, development of, 13

abortion, 47

adenocarcinoma in situ, 175

adenocarcinomas, breast cancer, 72

adenosquamous carcinoma, 170

adjuvant therapy, 126, 134, 143

age:
    breast cancer and, 9–10, 44
    ovarian cancer and, 209

alcohol consumption, breast cancer, 49–50

alpha fetoprotein (AFP) levels, 213

American Academy of Family Practice, 25

American Board of Radiologists, 120

American Cancer Society:
    I Can Cope program, 249
    publications, 245–47
    Reach to Recovery program, 110
    recommendations/guidelines:
        breast cancer detection, 230
        diet, nutrition, and cancer prevention, 51
        lymphedema, prevention strategies, 106
        for mammography, 24
        screening tests, 235–36
        silicone implants and, 111

American College of Obstetrics and American Gynecology, 24

American College of Physicians, 25

American Joint Committee on Cancer (AJCC), 77, 168, 213

American Medical Association, 25

American Society of Radiology, 25

anesthesia:
  breast-conserving treatment
    (BCT), 91
  cone biopsy, 165
  laparoscopy, 218
  mastectomy, 96
aneuploid cells, 75
angiogenesis, 76
angiosarcoma, 72
aspiration biopsy, 190
asymmetry, breast implants,
    113
atypical hyperplasia, 45
atypical squamous cells of
    undetermined significance
    (ASCUS), 155
autologous reconstruction:
  complications and side effects
    of, 118
  free flap, 117
  gluteus flap, 117
  latissimus dorsi flap, 114–15
  TRAM flap, 115–17
AutoPap, 155
axillary lymph nodes:
  breast cancer and, 21, 78, 84
  dissection, 93
axillary radiation therapy, 125

B

barium enema, 15
basal layer of uterus, 184
Bethesda System (TBS)
    Classifications, 156–57
bilateral salpingo-oophorectomy
    (BSO), 173, 197, 200, 219

biopsy:
  breast cancer diagnosis, 54–55,
    58–65
  cervical cancer, 163–64
  cone, 164–65
  core needle, 61–62
  defined, 55
  directed, 164–65
  endometrial, 189–91
  fine-needle aspiration biopsy
    (FNAB), 59–61
  mammography and, 24
  open, 63–65
  punch, 163–65
  purpose of, generally, 58–59
  sentinel lymph node, 95
  stereotactic, 62–63
birth control pills, 47–48, 160, 188
bladder, after radiation therapy,
    174
bleeding:
  abnormal, 10
  after biopsy, 164–65
  after mastectomy, 99–100
bleomycin, 175
bloating, 10, 12, 215
blood count, low, 139–40
body weight, breast cancer and,
    49. See also Obesity
bone marrow stem cells, 227
bone marrow transplant (BMT),
    131
brachytherapy, 173, 176, 198
BRCA 1/BRCA 2 gene(s), 41–43,
    208
breast, generally:
  anatomy of, 20–21

cancer of, *see* breast cancer
changes throughout life, 22–24, 46
clinical examination (CBE), 29–30
development of, 20–21
hormones and, 19–21
mammography, 24–29, 55–57
self-examination, 29–35
breast cancer:
cancer type, 72–73
chemotherapy:
    purpose of, generally, 16
    radiation therapy with, 127
    side effects of, 135–41
    stages of cancer, 141–44
    survival rate, 144
    who is helped by, 134–41
death rate, 7
defined, generally, 36
detection, 55
diagnosis, procedures, 66–85
diagnostic tools, 52–65
disease-fighting mechanisms, 40
early detection, 30
historical perspective, 126
incidence of, 7–9
information resources, 250–51
invasive, 38–39
pregnancy and, 92
preventive strategies, 50–51
recurrence of, 16, 89
research studies, 126–27
risk factors:
    generally, 9–10, 41–42

inherited, 42–45
lifestyle, 46–51
staging, 66, 141–44
surgery, *see* breast surgery
survival rate, 52
treatment options:
    chemotherapy, 126–44
    generally, 15–16, 81–84
    radiation therapy, 119–25
    stages of cancer, 141–44
    surgery, 67, 86–118
tumor grade, 73–74
breast-conserving treatment (BCT):
candidacy for, 90
procedure, overview, 90–92
ruling out conditions, 92–93
success rates, 89
breast feeding, 23
breast reconstruction surgery:
autologous, 114–18
nipple-areola, 118
timing of, 110–11
breast self-examination (BSE):
American Cancer Society's recommendations for, 30
importance of, 14, 30–31, 54
procedures, 32–35
breast surgeon:
fine-needle aspiration biopsy (FNAB), 61
implant procedures, 110–13
mastectomy procedures, 97
open biopsy, 63–65
selection of, 54–55
breast surgery:
breast-conserving, 87, 89–93

breast surgery (*cont.*)
  complications and side effects
      of, 99–107
  implants, 111–14
  lymph node dissection, 93–95
  mastectomy, 87–89, 96–99
  reconstruction, 108–10,
      114–18
  types of, generally, 87–89

C

CA, 129
CA-125, 192, 213, 234
CAF, 129
cancer type, determination of,
      72–73
capecitabine, 132
capsular contraction, 114
carcinoembryonic antigen
      (CEA), 213
carcinoma, defined, 36
carcinoma in situ:
  breast cancer, 70–71
  cervical cancer, 175–76
  treatment of, 175–76
cauterization, 165
cell division, 13
cell replication, 37–38
cell reproduction, 13
cervical canal, 147
cervical cancer:
  development of, 150
  diagnosis of, 167–70
  early-stage, 174
  incidence of, 12
  invasive, 12

mortality rates, 12
precancerous conditions,
      162–66
pregnancy in, 178
preinvasive, 12
risk factors, generally, 158–61
staging, 169
treatment options:
  chemotherapy, 174–75
  radiation therapy, 173–74,
      177, 179
  stage of cancer and, 175–79
  surgery, 172–73
types of, 168–70
cervicography, 163
cervix:
  abnormal cells, 16
  anatomy of, 147–48
  screening methods:
    Bethesda System (TBS)
        Classifications, 156–57
    Pap test, 149–55
checkups, importance of, 233–34
chemotherapy:
  breast cancer:
    commonly used drug
        combinations, 129–32
    generally, 75, 83–84, 95
    hormone therapy, 132–34
    how it works, 128–34
  cervical cancer, 174–75
  continuous infusion, 130–31
  endometrial cancer, 199–200
  ovarian cancer, 226–28
CIN (cervical intraepithelial
      neoplasia), 157, 166–67
cisplatin, 175

clear cell adenocarcinoma, 161
clinical breast examination
(CBE), 29–31, 54
Clinical Laboratory Improvement
Act (CLIA), 154
clinical staging, 76
clinical trials, 243–44
CMF, 129–30
colon cancer, death rate, 7
colonoscopy, 14–15
colorectal cancers, 7, 217
color flow Doppler imaging, 212
colposcopy, 155, 157, 163
Comprehensive Cancer Centers,
55
computed tomography (CT), 77,
192, 216
cone biopsy, cervical cancer,
164–65, 175–76
consolidation treatment, 225
constipation, 12
continuous infusion
chemotherapy, 130–31
contraception, as risk factor,
47–48, 169, 188
Cooper's ligaments, 21
core needle biopsy, 61–62
corpus, 183
corpus luteum, 206
corticosteroids, 129
counseling and support groups,
information resources,
251–54
cryosurgery, 165
cyclophosphamide, 129
cyst(s):
in the breast, 45, 58

fine-needle aspiration biopsy
(FNAB) and, 60–61
ovarian cancer and, 205, 218
cytoreductive surgery, 225
cytosarcoma phyllodes, 72
cytoxan, 129

D

DDE, 50
death rates:
generally, 7
ovarian cancer, 11–12
debulking surgery, 225, 229
delayed reconstruction, 108
DES daughters, 161
diagnosis, see screening tests
biopsy, 14
for breast cancer, 53–54,
74–76
pelvic exams, 11
diagnostic tests, see specific types
of tests
diet:
American Cancer Society's
guidelines, 51
breast cancer and, 48–49
ovarian cancer and, 210–11
diethylstilbestrol (DES), 161
dilation and curettage (D & C),
191
diploid cells, 75
directed biopsy, 164
discharge, from nipple, 56
distant metastasis, breast cancer,
79
docetaxel, 130

dosage, radiation therapy, 121
ductal carcinoma in situ (DCIS),
    70–71, 78, 141–42
ductal carcinomas, 72

E

early detection:
    breast cancer, 30, 55
    significance of, 26
ectocervix, 149
ectopic pregnancy, 217
egg, 205
endocervical curettage (ECC),
    164
endocervix, 148–49
endocrine therapy, 132–34
endometrial adenocarcinoma,
    185
endometrial biopsy, 189–91
endometrial cancer:
    prevention of, 188
    recurrent, 202
    risk factors, 186–87
    screening tests, 189
    staging, 195
    tamoxifen and, 187
    treatment of, 197–202
endometrial hyperplasia,
    187–88
endometriosis, 217
endometrium:
    cancer of the, 10–11
    defined, 184
environmental influences:
    breast cancer, 8, 44, 48, 50
    ovarian cancer, 161

epidermal growth factor, 76
epithelial cancer, 193
epithelial cells:
    in the breast, 21, 36, 45
    endometrial, 184
estrogen receptors (ER), 74
estrogen replacement therapy
    (ERT), 47, 188, 208
excisional biopsy, 63–64
exercise:
    after mastectomy, 100–104
    as prevention strategy, 49
    relaxation, 137
external beam radiation therapy,
    173, 176, 226
extraovarian serous carcinoma,
    209
extrusion, breast implants,
    113

F

fallopian tube, 183
false-negative Pap test, 153
false-positive Pap test, 153
familial breast cancer, 9, 42–45
family history, breast cancer in, 9,
    42–43
family support, information
    resources, 254–55
fatigue, from chemotherapy,
    138
fat necrosis, 56
fecal occult blood test, 14
fertility, ovarian cancer and,
    207
fibroadenoma, 56

financial issues, information resources, 263
fine-needle aspiration biopsy (FNAB), 59–61
5-fluorouracil (5-FU), 129, 132, 175
flow cytometry, 75
fluid buildup, after mastectomy, 99–103
follicles, 205
follicle-stimulating hormone (FSH), 22, 205
follow-up testing:
  mammography, 235
  Pap test, 234–35
  pelvic examination, 234–35
Food and Drug Administration (FDA), 111, 154–55
functional layer, of uterus, 184

G

gene(s):
  mutations:
    breast cancer, 43–44
    ovarian cancer, 208–209
  tumor suppression, 43
genetics:
  breast cancer and, 9, 42–43
  ovarian cancer and, 208–209
genital herpes virus, 159
genital sprays, 210
germinal epithelial, 205
glands, in the breast, 36
gonadotropin-releasing hormone, 205

gray, radiation therapy, 121
gynecologic cancers, information resources, 257–60

H

hair loss:
  chemotherapy, 135–36
  radiation therapy, 125
heart, chemotherapy effects on, 141
HER-2/neu, 76
herceptin, 76
hereditary nonpolyposis colon cancer (HNCC), 187
hereditary nonpolyposis colorectal cancer (HNPCC), 209
high-dose chemotherapy, 131, 144
high-fat diet, effects of, 48–49, 186, 210–11
histologic tumor grade, 73–74
home health care, information resources, 260–61
hormone receptors, 74
hormone replacement therapy, 23, 47
hormones, function of, 19–21
hormone therapy:
  breast cancer and, 84
  chemotherapy, 132–34
  ovarian cancer, 207–208
Hospice and supportive services, information resources, 261–62
hospitalization, mastectomy, 98

human chorionic gonadotropin (HCG), 213
human immunodeficiency virus (HIV), 159, 161
human papilloma virus (HPV), 150, 158
hyperplasia, 45
hysterectomy, *see specific types of hysterectomies*
    cervical cancer and, 151, 175
    as treatment option, generally, 16
hysteroscopy, 191

I

ifosfamide, 175
immediate reconstruction, 108
implants:
    complications and side effects of, 113–14
    surgery, 112–13
    types of, 111–12
incidence rates, generally, 6–9
incisional biopsy, 63–64
index, of cancer cells, 75
infection, after breast surgery, 107
inflammatory breast cancer, 72–73
information resources, generally, 255–57
informed consent, 60
insurance:
    coverage for breast reconstruction, 110
    information resources, 263
internal mammary nodes, 78

International Federation of Gynecology and Obstetrics (FIGO), 168, 196, 220
intraperitoneal P-32 radiation therapy, 226
intravenous pyelogram (IVP), 192
ipsilateral lymph nodes, 79

L

lactation, 23
laparoscope, 194
laparoscopy, 218–19
laparotomy, 219–20
laser surgery, 175
LEEP (loop electrosurgical excision procedure), 165–66, 172–73, 175
leukemia, 141
lifestyle risk factors:
    breast cancer, 46–51
    ovarian cancer, 210–11
lobular carcinoma in situ (LCIS), 45, 70, 78, 141–42
lobular carcinomas, 72
lobular neoplasia, 70
lobules, 21, 45
local control, 127
lumpectomy:
    diagnosis and, 15, 45
    re-excision, 92
    stage of cancer and, 142–43
lumps, in breast, 29, 31
lung cancer, death rate, 7
luteinizing hormone (LH), 22–23
lymphadenectomy, 93, 173, 177

lymphatic vessels, 21–22
lymphedema, 105–106, 125
lymph nodes:
   function of, 14, 21
   dissection, 93–95
   lymphedema, 105–106, 125
   mapping, 95
   metastatic cancer and, 77
   in pelvis, 148
   regional, 78–79
   status of, 135
Lynch Syndrome II, 209

M

magnetic resonance imaging
      (MRI), 77, 192, 216
malignant cells, metastasis, 13
mammary glands, 21
mammary ligaments, 21
mammatome, 62
mammogram:
   diagnostic, 53, 55–57
   reading, 56–57
mammography:
   American Cancer Society's
      recommendations,
      24, 29
   benefits of, 8, 14
   controversy over
      recommendations, 25
   defined, 24
   detection, American Cancer
      Society guidelines for, 29
   failure rate, 25
   follow-up testing, 235
   preparation for, 27

   procedure, overview, 27–28
   recordkeeping, 28–29
mastectomy:
   complications and side effects,
      99–107
   early discharge, 98
   emotional impact of, 85
   exercises recommended after,
      100–104
   modified radical, 88–89, 97
   partial, 87
   procedure, overview, 96–99
   purpose of, generally, 96
   radical, 89, 97
   reconstructive surgery and, 98,
      108–10
   segmental, 87
   simple, 88
   subcutaneous, 88
   total, 88
   as treatment option, 59, 67
medical oncologist, 127–28
medullary breast cancer, 72
menarche, age at onset, 46. *See
      also* menstruation
menopause:
   age at onset, 186–87
   breast cancer and, 18, 23–24,
      46, 55
   chemotherapy and, 132, 140
   uterine cancer and, 186–87
menstruation:
   breast changes, 22–23
   cervical cancer and, 173
   changes in cycle, 236
   uterine cancer and, 185
methotrexate, 129

microcalcifications, in breast, 56
micrometastases, 126
milk sinuses, 21
miscarriage, 47, 207
modified radical mastectomy, 88–89, 97
mortality rates, 6–7, 12
mother:
    breast cancer in, 9
    ovarian cancer in, 11
mucinous breast cancer, 72
myometrium, 184

N

National Cancer Institute:
    American Cancer Society Breast Cancer Detection Demonstration Project, 27
    Physicians Data Query (PDQ), 80
    research studies, generally, 55, 89
National Institute of Health, 214
National Medical Association, 25
National Surgical Adjuvant Breast Protocol (NSABP), 94
nausea, 12, 136–37
neoadjuvant therapy, 126–27, 144
nipple-areola reconstruction, 118
nitrosamines, 159–60
nolvadex, 16
nuclear grade, 73

nutrition, see diet
    aging and, 9
    cervical cancer and, 160
    significance of, 40

O

obesity, as risk factor, 186
omentum, 194, 222
one-step procedure, 59, 77
oocyte, 205
oophorectomy, 132
open biopsy, 63–65
oral cavity, cancer in, 14
oral contraception, as risk factor, 47–48, 169, 188
os, 148
ovarian ablation, 132
ovarian cancer:
    defined, 215
    diagnostic surgery, 217–20
    early stage, 219
    experimental therapy, 231
    incidence of, 10
    mortality rates, 11–12
    recurrent, 227, 230–31
    risk factors, 206–11
    screening tests, 211–14
    staging, 220–22
    survival rate, 12, 229
    symptoms, 12, 215
    treatment options:
        chemotherapy, 226–28
        radiation therapy, 226
        stage of cancer and, 228–30
        surgery, 224–25

tumors:
  detection, 216–17
  of low malignant potential,
    231
  types of, 220
ovaries, anatomy of, 205–206
ovulation, 205

P

paclitaxel, 130, 200
Paget's disease, 78
pain:
  abdominal, 10–11
  after breast surgery, 106–107
  management, information
    resources, 263
pancreatic cancer, death rate, 7
Papanicolaou, George, Dr.,
    149
PAPNET, 155
pap test:
  accuracy of, 153–55
  American Cancer Society's
    recommendations for,
    150–51
  development of, 149
  follow-up testing, 234–35
  preparation for, 152
  procedure, generally, 151, 153
  purpose of, 11, 15, 149–50
partial hysterectomy, 151
partial mastectomy, 87
pathologic staging, 76
pathologist:
  malignancy, determination by,
    69, 71–72

open biopsy, 64
role of, generally, 58
pathology report, breast cancer,
    71
patient records, importance of,
    81–82
PCBs, 50
pelvic examination:
  follow-up testing, 234–35
  importance of, 11–12, 15
peripheral blood stem cells, 227
peritoneal papillary serous
    carcinoma, 209
peritoneum, 193
p53 genes, 43–44
ploidy, of cancer cells, 75
positron-emission tomography
    (PET), 216
predisposing factors, genetics, 9,
    42–43, 208–209
prednisone, 129
pregnancy:
  breast cancer and, 47, 92
  cervical cancer, 178
  ectopic, 217
  maternal age and, 8–9
  ovarian cancer and, 207
preoperative chemotherapy, 127
preventive strategies, breast
    cancer, 50–51
primary tumor, 16, 77–78
progesterone, uterine cancer and,
    186
progesterone receptors (PR), 74
prognostic factors, breast cancer,
    69
prophylactic oophorectomy, 209

prostate cancer, death rate, 7
puberty:
    breast development, 20–21
    menstruation, *see* menarche;
        menstruation
punch biopsy, 163–64

Q

quadrantectomy, 87

R

radiation nurses, 120
radiation oncologist, 120–21
radiation team, functions of, 120
radiation technologists, 120
radiation therapy:
    breast cancer:
        basics of, 121
        chemotherapy with, 127
        preparation for, 121–23
        side effects, 124
        stages of cancer, 142, 144
        time frame, 122
        as treatment option,
            generally, 16, 83, 120
        weekly treatments, 123–25
    cervical cancer:
        side effects, 174
        as treatment option,
            generally, 177, 179
        types of, 173–74
    endometrial cancer, 197–99,
        202
radiation treatment, *see* radiation
    therapy

radical mastectomy, 89, 97
radiologist, role of, 56–57
reconstructive surgery, *see* breast
    reconstruction surgery
rectal cancer, 7
rectal exam, 15
recurrent cancer, 202, 227
re-excision lumpectomy, 92
regional control, 84, 127
relatives:
    first-degree, 9, 44, 209
    third-degree, 44
remission, breast cancer, 130
reproductive organs, cancers of,
        *see specific reproductive
        organs*
research, diagnostic testing, 75–76
risk factors,
    breast cancer, 9–10, 41–51
    endometrial cancer, 186–87
    ovarian cancer, 206–11

S

saline infusion sonogram, 192
screening tests:
    breast cancer, 8, 14
    colon cancer, 14
    general cancer-related
        checkups, 14
    ovarian cancer:
        generally, 12
        tumor markers, 213–14
        ultrasonography, 211–13
    rectal cancer, 14–15
second-look laparotomy, 225, 230
second-look surgery, 225

second opinions, 57, 66, 68–69, 81, 83

secretions, from breast, 35, 56

segmental mastectomy, 87

self-exams, importance of, 236. *See also* breast self-examination (BSE)

sensitivity, after breast surgery, 107

sentinel lymph node biopsy, 95

seroma, 100

serosa, 184

sexual behavior, cervical cancer and, 158–59

sexual intercourse, restricted, 165, 174

sexually transmitted disease (STD), 158–59

sigmoidoscopy, 14

SIL (low/high-grade squamous cell abnormalities), 157–58

silicone-gel implants, 111

simple hyperplasia, 188

simple hysterectomy, 172–73, 200

simple mastectomy, 88

simulator, radiation therapy, 121

sisters:
    breast cancer in, 9, 45
    ovarian cancer in, 11

skin cancer, 8, 14

Skin Cancer Foundation, 236

small cell carcinomas, 170

social support, importance of, 67–68, 124

sonogram, *see* ultrasonography

s-phase fraction, 75

squamous cell carcinomas, 72, 170

staging:
    breast cancer, 66, 76–80
    cervical cancer, 169, 176–77, 179
    endometrial cancer, 195
    uterine cancer, 193–94

stereotactic biopsy, 62–63

sternum, 21

stomal sarcomas, 193

stress reduction strategies, 238

subcutaneous mastectomy, 88

subtotal hysterectomy, 151

suction biopsy, *see* fine-needle aspiration biopsy (FNAB)

surgery:
    breast, *see* breast surgery
    cervical cancer, 172–73
    one-step procedure, 59, 77
    as treatment, generally, 13
    two-step procedure, 59, 77
    uterine cancer, 193–94

survival rates:
    breast cancer, 80, 144
    ovarian cancer, 12

survivors:
    lifestyle changes, 238–39
    quality of life, 241–42
    returning to work, 237–38
    sexuality and intimacy, 239–41

swelling, after breast surgery, 105–106

symptoms:
    cancer of the reproductive organs, generally, 10–11
    ovarian cancer, 12, 215

synthesis phase, 75
systemic control, 84, 127

T

talcum powder, 210
tamoxifen, 16, 132–34, 187, 200,
     234
taxol, 129–30
taxotere, 130
teletherapy, 173, 176
tenderness:
   abdominal, 10–11
   in breast, 21, 35
   after breast surgery, 107
ThinPrep, 154
thrombophlebitis, 134
thyroid cancer, 14
total hysterectomy, 151, 197, 219,
     229
total mastectomy, 88
transformation zone, 149, 151
transvaginal sonography (TVS),
     191, 211–13
tubal sterilization, 207
tubular breast cancer, 72
tumor(s):
   formation of, 13
   grade, in breast cancer, 73–74
   markers, 213–14
   removal options, 82–83
   suppressor genes, 43
two-step procedure, 59, 77

U

ultrahysterosonogram, 192
ultrasonography:
   breast cancer, 57–58

uterine cancer, 211–13
   vaginal, 211
United States Preventive Services
     Task Force, 25
usual hyperplasia, 45
uterine cancer:
   defined, 185–88
   diagnostic tests, 190–92
   endometrial cancer,
        prevention of, 188
   screening tests, 15, 189
   staging, generally, 194
   surgical staging, 193–94
   types of, 193
uterine sarcomas, 193
uterus, anatomy of, 183–85

V

vaginal hysterectomy, 194
vaginal ultrasound, 211
vitamin deficiencies, impact of,
     160

W

weight gain, from chemotherapy,
     138–39
white-cell count, 139
wire localization, 63

X

xeloda, 132

Y

YWCA, 264

About the Authors

CAROLYN D. RUNOWICZ, M.D., is a nationally prominent expert in the treatment of gynecologic cancers. She was selected as one of the leading oncologists by American Health Magazine, New York Magazine, and Best Doctors in America. She is Director of Gynecologic Oncology and Professor of Obstetrics and Gynecology at the Albert Einstein College of Medicine and Montefiore Medical Center, where she is in charge of education, research, and clinical practice.

JEANNE A. PETREK, M.D., is the Director of the Surgical Program of the Lauder Breast Center of Memorial Sloan Kettering Cancer Center. Well-known in the area of breast cancer research and treatment, she was also named by the New York Times in 1997 as one of the twelve leaders in women's health. Her research studies investigate the effect of breast cancer treatment on pre-menopausal women.

TED S. GANSLER, M.D., is the Director of Health Content at the American Cancer Society where he is responsible for assuring the accuracy of printed and electronic information products for patients and the public. He has taught and practiced pathology at Emory University and the Medical University of South Carolina.

DIANNE PARTIE LANGE has been a health writer and editor for twenty-five years. Her articles have appeared in *Allure, New Woman, Living Fit, The New York Times,* and *American Health.* Her health news column, *Body News,* has been a regular feature in *Allure* for six years. Most recently, she co-authored with Lois B. Morris and Dr. Gerald P. Murphy, *Informed Decisions: The American Cancer Society's Guide to Cancer Detection and Treatment and Recovery* (Viking, 1997). She is also a Registered Nurse.

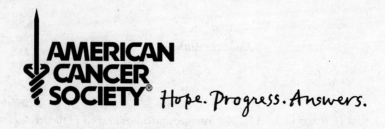

AMERICAN
CANCER
SOCIETY® Hope. Progress. Answers.

The American Cancer Society is the nationwide community-based voluntary health organization dedicated to eliminating cancer as a major health problem by preventing cancer, saving lives from cancer, and diminishing suffering from cancer through research, education, and service.

For information on cancer and on American Cancer Society educational programs and services, please contact:

Toll-free cancer information: 800-ACS-2345
Home page address: http://www.cancer.org